Sensational Motions

Stories to Exercise By

By Charlotte Saben

Sensational Motions: Stories to Exercise By
All rights reserved
September 24, 2016
Copyright ©2016 Charlotte Saben
ISBN-13: 978-1539072089
ISBN-10: 1539072088

Disclaimer

These movements are not meant to take the place of therapeutic exercise. **PLEASE** know your residents and their limitations. **ALWAYS** remind residents that although a little discomfort can be normal in movement, pain and soreness is **not** necessarily. Therefore, if it hurts**, DO NOT DO IT!!!** These are not meant to push the residents but rather to just get them moving and thinking.

If there are rehab or Restorative nursing residents, please check with therapist to make sure they are safe to participate. **Doctors' orders or approval may be required**. Please check with the appropriate managers to ensure the safety of your residents.

These movements or motions may be done from wheelchairs. Most of these motions are fairly gentle and easy, but some residents can still be at risk of falling from wheelchairs or sitting/standing positions. When using the words like "bent over" instruct them to lean gently in their chair rather than reach for their toes! **PLEASE USE CAUTION!**

PLEASE pre-read each story, not only to determine what sensory items you might like to produce, but also to evaluate which movements you want to use and what discussion to evoke.

Table of Contents

Sensational Motions is a new program bringing together exercise, reminiscing, and at least a few of the five senses. It is designed for populations within the skilled nursing, assisted living, memory care, and group home settings. It begins with the reading of one of 52 stories (that's one for each week, but you can use them more frequently.) They relate to the residents' current or past lives. There is humor and/or emotional triggers within each story. Each story has action words that the residents are cued to listen for while the leader reads the story initially. This gives them the chance to process the theme and enjoy the story as well as prepare themselves for the types of physical movement the story may request. Most movements (motions) can be done from a sitting position, including wheelchairs. This has been designed originally for long-term care facilities, SNF, but has been used in other settings successfully.

No one is required to do any of the exercises, but all are encouraged to do what they can. The leader re-reads the story, stopping at all the action words (which are in **bold type** in the story). The leader continues to relate the story's emotional/sensory questions as they continue the exercise movement. (These questions or thought provokers are in *italics and parenthesis* in the printed story). Then the residents begin to share a response, the repetitive movement is paused and discussion should ensue. Then, the leader picks up where they left off on the story and movement continues.

At the end of the story/exercise time, discussion is encouraged. Often sensory items are offered. A list of suggestions for this follows. The **leaders should pre-read the story prior to the group setting** so they understand the requests the story presents to their participants. Where there are ***bolded AND italicized*** words, these are not meant to be read, but are rather suggestions of actions or discussion thoughts. This is another reason for pre-reading the story!

There are certain on-going "themes" throughout the book. For example, when a situation occurs in which it would be natural for a person to swear (or cuss) the group "accentuates their vowels". This means they say each vowel-A-E-I-O-U loudly and with very wide mouth movements. They should discover that each vowel sound requires a different shape of the mouth, thus using various muscles. This occurs in many stories!

When there are rather ambiguous words or words that have more than one meaning, taking advantage of the meaning that evokes the most action is best. For example: such words as "hoped", "prayed", "approached", "moved", "poked", "cook", etc. can have varied motions from praying hands, "free movement" to whatever the reader/leader feels is appropriate. Even if the word is used as a noun, such as "the cook", the leader may suggest a stirring of the pot motion with wrists, or flipping of pancake motions, etc. Feel free to use your own imagination with those! When pre-reading the story, the leader may think of a fun movement or comment that is appropriate. If you do not feel that a given bolded word is appropriate movement for your population, do not use it. The residents will be caught up in the story and whatever motions the leader suggests.

There are some action words which are highlighted that, in themselves, are not appropriate action for most elder populations. These can be "dropped", "fell", "trip", "bend over", "jump", "scamper", etc. In this case, the leader suggests a simpler, safer movement such as bending slightly, pretending to drop something from the hand, moving feet in upward motion, etc. or you can just skip that action.

Action words such as "chat", "talk", "yell", "laugh", "sing", etc. can be mimicked with hand gestures or belly rubs, mouth movements or as leader sees fit. When "hug" is used, it is suggested that we hug ourselves and then again…with the opposite arm on top!

The words "sitting", "standing", etc. are used sparingly. If your population has the ability and agility to accomplish this, that is fine with supervision. However, in most cases, it would be best to either skip those words in the exercise portion of the story or choose hand motions representing those words. An opportunity for sign-language lessons exists here as well!

You will find certain stories that have controversial topic for conversation. Not all stories are humorous and light-hearted, but the questions lead to thought-provoking discussion. Also, there are some stories that are overly silly, perhaps seeming nonsensical. Please remember that these are written for a variety of populations; some with severe dementia as well as those who are cognitively sound. I tried to make all stories relatable to the majority of residents. If a particular story does not meet your population's criteria, please skip it or adapt as needed. I have no issues with adaptations, provided proper acknowledgement is due. Have fun and enjoy! I plan for more to be coming soon.

Charlotte Saben, ADC, AP-BC

1. Pre-read the story to determine which action words, discussion topics, and sensory items may be appropriate for your population.

2. Read the story by itself for the enjoyment of the story. Suggestion: Ask the residents to listen for the action words.

3. Read the story through again, demonstrating the action or exercise words, and reading the discussion questions or comments as they do the repetitive movements you are demonstrating. At the conclusion of reasonable amount of movement, the discussion can continue. Then continue on with the next phase of the story and repeat.

4. Present items for sensory integration. Try to include as many senses as possible but keep the items relevant to the story.

There is such a wide variety of opportunity here! I will give you some examples to guide the creative spirit within you!

For example, there is a story about a young lady riding her bike through the desert. At the end, you can pass around a small succulent and pictures of snakes and other desert dwellers. Offer tastes of honey or cactus jelly. Another story of a rodeo (suggested by residents) invokes a video of cows, horses, etc. along with the reminiscing. Things to taste and touch: Milk products, or rope or leather, suede, spurs, etc.) The mention of a bakery in a story might present a good time for coffee and donuts or baking bread in a bread machine!

A story of a walk on the beach: shells, sea stars, sand dollars, videos of ocean or surfing, etc. Webcams of beach resorts, sounds of waves crashing or sea gulls cawing; Taste of small bits of saltwater taffy (be careful of it sticking to dentures!) or salmon, etc.

Christmas, Holidays, snow themes: Pictures or videos of falling snow, skiing, etc. Fake snow can be touched or snow cones can be made and sampled for flavor or just for feel. Cocoa and cookies, Holiday music, smells of spices, etc.

Stuffed animals can be used in many stories. Postcards, pictures, etc. for things to see. Most libraries have CDs of sounds of birds, nature, etc.

These are just a few examples of the many sensory items that can accompany these stories, even leading into other groups. Imagine! Explore! Have fun! And by the way, these stories are just as enjoyable without the sensory items. I have sometimes used a story without them, and then re-used it a few weeks later with them and the residents thought it was all fresh and new! Enjoy!

Once there was a young woman. She loved to take **walk**s down by the seashore. She loved to watch the *waves* **roll** in and out. Sometimes seagulls would **scream** overhead and **swoop down** to snatch a wayward fish. *(Did you ever take a stroll on the beach? Where else did you like to walk?)*

That often startled her and she would **pick up the pace** and even **run** and **jog** a bit. Sometimes she would **kick** off her shoes and let the sand run through her toes. *(What does that feel like?)* She loved the smell of the beach. *(What did it smell like?)*

She followed the coastline, **marching** to the beat of the drummer in her head. *(How fast is your drummer?)*

She would arrive shortly at a small forest. She loved to feel the breeze and watch the trees **sway** back and forth. *(If you were a tree, what kind would you want to be?)*

She found a hollow log. She **sat** down on it and **rocked** back and forth. She knew it was hollow because when she **knocked** on it, there was a hollow sound. She so **rocked** on, **touching her knees and toes**, **shaking** the sand from the toes. She **rolled her ankles** to make sure the sand was gone.

She didn't realize that the sun was rapidly setting. The moon **peeked** out from behind the clouds. *(Have you ever seen shapes in the clouds? Can you tell me about them, and even draw them with your hand?)*

She hoped she could **reach** for the stars and **pluck** one out of the sky. She **hummed** a little song about that. *(Can you remember a song about stars? Let's sing it!)*

She decided to **draw** in the sand. The forest was full of sand and clay. She **stirred** with a stick, designing a big circle representing the setting sun. She **stretched her arms** to **make circles** so she could be stronger. **Stirring** in the clay can be hard! *(Have you watched a beautiful sunset? Where were you and who were you with?)*

She **kicked** at a rock that dared to intrude on her circle. She **clapped her hands** to scare away a squirrel, because she was afraid of squirrels. *(Are you afraid of any animals? What are you afraid of?)*

Touching each finger to her thumb, she **pushed** herself up off the rock. She knew she had to get home quickly. What was the best way to cross the river? She could **swim**. She could **wade.** OR she could **walk** over the bridge. (*Which one would you choose?*)

She finally made it to the street where she lived. She gave herself and her family a big **hug.** She even **patted herself on the back**! She made it home before dark! She **reached** into her pocket. And she **made a face!** She made a *happy face*. She made a *sad face*. She made a *disgusted face.* She made a *smiley face*. She even **stuck out her tongue**! And then she swore! Not really, she just **accentuated her vowel sounds**! That was her way of swearing! She **reached** into her pocket again! What is that? Did she indeed **catch** a star? Or was it a starfish? You decide!

Charlotte Saben, ADC, AP-BC

Once there was a handsome old gent. He liked to go for a long leisurely **walk** each day. He started out by **bending to touch his toes.** Then he **pulled** his boots onto his feet and **stomped** out of the house. He **walked.** He came to the lumber yard where he watched the men **saw back and forth** on a big board. He wanted to try it too, but they wouldn't let him. *(Have you ever sawn a board with a blade saw?)*

He **walked** on further. He passed the bakery. Boy! That bread smells good! *(What is your favorite kind of bread? What is your favorite bakery item?)* He mimicked the baker **rolling** the dough and **kneading** it. He **laughed** a big belly-laugh, **heaving and rolling his shoulders.** He pretended to **toss** a pizza into the air, even though bakeries usually don't make pizza! He **made faces** in the window. He knew the owner very well. Big Sam would make a face right back at him. And then they would **wave** goodbye. *(What does a bakery smell like?)*

He passed the park. He wanted to stop, but knew he must get home before lunch because his wife had made his favorite dish. He knew because he had watched her **tossing the salad**, **peeling** the carrots, **stirring** the pot, and **licking** her fingers. **(We won't lick our fingers today, but we can exercise them by touching each one to the thumb.)** She always **shook her hands** dry because she hated washing towels. *(What is the household chore you disliked the most? What was your favorite?)*

A dog **ran** out from the park and **barked** at him. He began to **run**. He **clicked** his **heels and then his toes** as he **sauntered** down the lane. He finally hid behind a tree. A nice breeze made them **sway**. *(What kinds of trees were there on the property where you grew up? How about where you raised your family?)* He wished it was an apple tree so he could **pick** some!

Then he passed the newspaper van. He remembered delivering papers when he was a boy. He had **ridden a bicycle** to do it back then. Now they just **drive** by in a car and **fling** the paper with their arms. He **stretched** out his arms and **made circles, starting with a tiny one, then bigger, and bigger still!** He was quite certain he was still stronger than the person he just saw tossing papers. *Have you ever had a paper route? What did you use to get around in? How many did you deliver each day?*

He rounded the bend **stepping high.** The ice cream truck caught his eye! He knew he should just ignore it and eat his wife's lovely lunch…BUT!

He **opened his mouth** wide. Would he **yawn**? Would he **eat** an ice cream? *(Show me what YOU would do!)*

He finally came to his own front yard. He **swung** the gate open, and **shuffled** up the sidewalk. But he was late for lunch! He thought perhaps his wife would not give him a hug, so he **hugged** himself! Not once, but SIX times! And then he **patted** himself on the back! After all, he HAD made it home!

He **opened** the door, **looked to the right, left, and up and down!** Then he **smiled**.

His wife was sitting at the table waiting patiently for him. Well, maybe NOT so patiently, as he could see the dog licking his nozzle and the cat licking her paws. *(Do you think there was any lunch left for him? What would you do if your spouse was late?)* ***(Could also reminisce about pets you've had, or arguments over food, being late, etc.)***

Charlotte Saben, ADC, AP-BC

It is raining. It is pouring. And Tom must **step over** and **splash through** the puddles. He also **opens** his umbrella and **twirls it in the air, waving** it as if the wind itself was capturing it. He actually did almost blow away. Better be careful, Tom! (*Did you ever go splashing through the puddles as a kid? How about as an adult? Would you if you could and no one was watching?*)

He **ran** into the mall to get out of the rain. He **pulled** the umbrella close to his chest and **folded** it in his arms, **hugging himself** in the process. He wished he hadn't decided to go shopping today. (*Have you ever picked a bad-weather day to do something? Did you get stuck in a storm? What did it sound, feel, smell, etc, like? What did you do?*)

But, alas! He had indeed! He sat down on the bench, **bending** carefully at the waist and **shook** the water off **his feet.** He **rolled his ankles** to be sure his socks were not too wet! He **touched his toes** several times just to see if he could! It felt good to sit after all that splashing and **high stepping**. He **took a deep breath**, in and out. He loved the smell of the rain, even if it was mixed with other smells. (*What does rain smell like to you? What other smells could have been mixed in? What is your favorite smell?*)

He **stretched his arms above his head** like a sprawling cat! He **yawned** like one too! He **opened and shut his hands** several times because the dampness made his arthritis act up! His **fingers stretched** out, practically on their own! He dreamed of the fire in the hearth at home. He found himself **making crackling sounds and motions!** What a silly guy! (*Do you like having a fire in the fireplace? What about a campfire? What memories do you have sitting around a fire?*)

He realized that people were looking at him strangely. And some of them were **holding their hands over their ears!** He must be making those sounds louder than he thought! OOPS! (*Would you like to share an embarrassing moment you had, or saw someone else do, in public?*)

He **turned his head to the right and then to the left**. He **looked up and down**. He **rolled his neck in both directions**, trying to clear his thoughts. How would he get out of this embarrassing moment? He **kicked** at the sidewalk and **stood** to his feet. (If you can't stand, **bend slightly forward**, placing your hands on your legs. **Push yourself back into the straight sitting position using your arm power!**)

"Look at that will you!?" He declared, **looking up** to the sky. He **made faces**. First he **puckered** like he was going to whistle. (*Can you whistle? Did you whistle as a kid? Did you have wooden or plastic whistles? What did you whistle at?*)

Then he **blew a kiss** into the air! And he **turned his head** with a **pout**! He **scowled**. He **raised his eyebrows**! He **made a mean face**. He **made a mad face**. Then he **smiled broadly** and **laughed** out loud. "Gottcha!" He said. There was nothing in the sky to see other than the clouds and a few birds. (*Do you like birds? What kinds of birds do you like? If you could be a bird, what bird would you be? What would you look like?* **OR** *tell me about shapes you have seen in clouds. What would you see if you were floating on a cloud?*)

Tom continued to **laugh** as he **shuffled** down the sidewalk, **stepping right and then left.** The rain had stopped and a beautiful rainbow arched the sky. NOW there was something to **look up** at, indeed! This made Tom's feet **dance** so he **two stepped it** back to the parking lot. (*Tell me about a time you saw a rainbow. What did it mean to you? How did it make you feel?*) He **opened his car door** and **climbed** in. He **drove** (make steering motions and feet pedal motions) too rapidly down the street, splashing pedestrians as he went by…still **laughing**! What an adventure he had! (*Was Tom being a good guy or a bad guy with his splashing? Have you ever driven too fast in the rain? How would you drive in a storm?*)

Tom managed to arrive home safely and **gave himself a big hug**! He had totally forgotten to do his shopping after all! But he had quite an adventure so all ended happily…except maybe for those pedestrians he drenched!

Charlotte Saben, ADC, AP-BC

Darlene **slammed** the trunk down and **opened** the car door. She **climbed** inside and **turned** the key. She **twisted her wrist** and **shook her hands** and **opened and closed them** several times. She was excited to start this new bowling team. But it had been half a decade at least since she belonged to one. *(Did you ever bowl on a team?)*

Nancy **ran** up beside the car. "Did you forget me?" she yelled, **half laughing**! Darlene **looked down**. She *had* forgotten about Nancy, but she didn't want to admit it. She **looked up** at the sky.

"Looks like a good day to be inside…so get in!"

Nancy **looked up too and then down** again. She **looked to the left and then the right**. She **made rolling motions with her hands**.

"What are you doing?" asked Darlene as she **rolled her neck around** to release her stress. She hated it when she forgot things…much more so when it's people!

"Just **rolling** with the clouds!" explained Nancy. "Thought I'd **stretch my arms** a bit before the big game!"

"Now you sound like some jock! 'Before the big game' indeed! You haven't **bowled** in longer than me! More like a big joke!"

Nancy didn't reply but **rolled her ankles** round and round. She **tapped her feet** to the rhythm of the music on the radio. *(What song was on the radio? Let's sing a song and tap to it to!)* Darlene was a good friend, but sometimes she just must remind us of things we want to forget! And sometimes she forgets things she should remember!

"By the way, the last time we went **bowling** you…" Darlene started to reminisce.

"That's quite enough, thank you!" Nancy retorted. She remembered all right! She had **stepped** up to the line, **brought the ball back**, then heard the "thud!". How embarrassing that the ball landed behind her! But worse yet, she had **crisscrossed her legs**, trying to keep from falling. She must have looked like a drunken sailor needing to find a bathroom! Then she had **bent over** to retrieve the ball, and **stepped** on her untied shoelace! *(Would you feel embarrassed?) (Have you ever had a gaffe during a public sport?)*

She **shuddered** at the memory! Won't let that happen again! She **bent down** in the car to make sure her laces were tied. She **shook her feet** and then **her hands.**

Darlene **gripped** the wheel and **pushed down** on the accelerator!

Nancy **hugged** herself and **made a face**. She didn't particularly like the way Darlene **drove**. But, she loved the thought of reuniting her bowling team, so she **closed her eyes and pretended to be somewhere else.** *(Where would you go if you went to your favorite place on earth?) (What would it sound, smell, look, feel like?) (Do you have a friend whose driving scares you? Or a friend who was scared of your driving?)*

She saw herself **walking** along the beach, **smelling** the salty air. She imagined she held a seashell in her hand. She **opened and closed them several times** and **pressed each finger to the thumb**. She felt a squishy liquid on her hand. *(What do you think that was?)*

Suddenly she awoke to the **screeching** of tires and a sudden jolt. She **opened the door** and **ran** inside. Darlene was right behind her, trying to remember what she had forgotten. It seemed like there was something special about today. She **scratched her head** and then **shook it.** Darlene noticed everyone was **smiling…** in a very sly way.

"Surprise! Happy Birthday, Darlene!" they said in unison and then **sang** the familiar song to her. *(Sing! What other songs might you sing for a birthday?)*

Darlene had more fun than ever before; with cake on her face…she **wiped** it several times. She **blew kisses** to all her teammates as she sent the ball down the lane. *(**Make bowling motions**).* It was a good day after all! Sometimes forgetting isn't so bad! It can lead to surprises!

Charlotte Saben, ADC, AP-BC

She **rolled her shoulders forwards and then backwards** and then **rotating**. She did a little **bounce on her seat**. The bumpy road made her **move up and down** like a jumping bean. The cactus seemed to fly by. This bike ride in the desert was more than she had expected. And less too. *(What would you expect to see if you were riding a bicycle in the desert? What would the desert feel like? Smell like? Sound like?)* She **pedaled** faster, with the dirt flying up in her face. She **made a face; a squinty face; then she rolled her lips around almost touching her nose!** Maybe that will keep the dust and bugs out of her face!

She **pedaled** past the roadrunner, although he passed her up shortly. She slowed and then stopped at the oasis. She **hopped** off her bike and **ran** to the shade cover. She **kicked** at the bike rest trying to make it support her bike. She took several **deep breaths in and out**. She **heaved her chest**, taking in the scenes around her. *(What scenes make you relax? Tell us about a special place you'd love to be!)*

She **bent down** to tie her shoelace which had worked itself undone. She **shook her feet** and **moved her ankles in circles** to improve the blood flow. What a ride it was so far! Dodging cacti was not so much fun. *(Where would you prefer to ride your bike? Have you ever had a cactus garden? Tell me about it.)*

She **walked** to the fountain and **splashed** the cool water on her face, and **slapped** some on **her back**. She **shook her wrists** vigorously from the tight grip of the handlebars. She **opened and shut her hands** several times to loosen the muscles. *(Have you ever been very thirsty with limited water? How did you feel when you found some? What did the water feel, taste, smell, etc. like to you then?)*

She **stretched her arms above her head, and swayed** like a tree. **Clasping her fingers together with her arms above her head, she made a full circle and back** the other way. This helped **stretch her muscles** and clear her mind at the same time! What a beautiful sight this desert was. Not barren at all! She admitted, though, that it was full of creepy crawly critters she did not want to embrace. She **stretched out her arms to embrace the air and her**self. She gave herself a big bear **hug!** She deserved it. *(Tell me why you deserve a big bear hug!)*

She took another **deep breath,** in through the nose *(what might she smell?)* and out through the mouth! She **climbed** on her bike again with **big strides**. And then she **jumped** off again!

She **bent** again to **touch her toes** and **stretch** her back. She **looked up** to the sky. A big hawk soared above and cawed loudly as if mocking her. She mimicked the bird, **spreading her arms out as if flying**…no, soaring through the air! She also mocked his sounds. How silly that felt! (*What might you see if you were a bird? What kind of bird would you want to be if you had to be a bird? What would a bird eat in the desert?*) **She rolled her neck**, noticing some small pebbles on a bench. She **picked** them up and **tossed** them into the air.

A pair of quail **ran** out of the bushes when the pebbles landed in their bush home. She **picked up** a larger rock which was lying by the bench. It was heavier than she had thought. She **pulled** it up, though, until she had it in her hand like a weight. She **threw** it with a **mighty heave**. The rock made a loud sound when it the ground and the dust flew! She **made a face with her mouth** as the dust permeated her throat. She didn't even know why she thought she needed to throw that rock in the first place! (*Have you ever done something spontaneous and didn't even know why?*)

The girl got back on her bike and **pedaled** once again. It wasn't long until she **saw** the station ahead. **(*Pretend you are looking…place hand on forehead and turn head side to side*).** She **pedaled** faster. The wheels of the bike were **spinning** rapidly as the tires bounced along. **(*Make spinning motions with hands*)**

Her adventure was complete! She had made it safely through the desert. Now she would **sit down** and **write** about it on her Tablet. She **thumbed** through the pictures on her phone, selecting a few to confirm her adventure. These would find their way to her social media for bragging rights! (*Tell me something you can brag about! Do you use social media?*)

Tom **walked slowly** down the dusty path. He remembered the days when he **ran** out to this same field, ready to **throw the football**. He wanted to **kick** the dirt, but was afraid he might fall. He heard his keys **drop** to the ground and **bent** to pick them up. He **flexed his fingers** and **brought each of them individually to his thumb**. Then he **opened and closed his hands** several times. Arthritis was not going to stop him from **watching** his grandson play soccer or from **picking up** those keys! *(Move hands to eyes as if looking for something. Bring them down again. Repeat several times.)*

Soccer seemed to be the sport of the day. Football was too rough for the kids these days. Tom didn't think that was true, but most of the parents did. "Kids just can't take any criticism, roughness, or real competition." Tom thought to himself. He **swatted** at a fly who dared to cross his face. *(What sports did you play as a kid? How about your children/grandchildren? What do you think about competition for children in sports…how should it be handled?)*

He **unfolded** his lawn chair and **tapped his feet** to make sure the dirt wasn't loose. Then he **stomped** a few times and **drew a good luck symbol in the dirt with the toe of his shoe.** He **sat** down. This would be a good day. He could tell because his neck was flexible and he could **roll** it around easily. That was always a good day. He **looked to the right and then to the left** trying to find his pride and joy, Justin. *(Tell me about your grandchildren…)*

There he was! His bright red shirt and yellow socks made him stand out. The rest of his team had red shirts, but the yellow socks were uniquely his. It was a long story and Tom had forgotten most of it. All he remembered was that Justin ended up with the yellow socks…and there was a funny reason for it.

He **stretched his arms in the air and above his head.** Might as well practice cheering. He **pumped his arms** to show his muscle…the same kind Justin had inherited. He **grabbed** at the flies swarming the air. He cursed under his breath, but loud enough that his son heard him. "Dad! None of that! **Accentuate your vowels** if you must say something like that!" Tom hated **pronouncing his vowels with wide mouthed movements,** but he had agreed to that over swearing. He **moved his arms in circles** and **rotated his wrists**, as if writing a protest.

Justin **ran** out onto the field with his team. He **crisscrossed his feet** as he moved the ball down the field. He **kicked it sideways, swinging his feet wide**. His teammate **slid** the ball past the goalie for a goal! Yes, Sir! This is a good day!

But Tom **made a face** at the next play. The other team head-butted the ball over the goal post and it **hit** a bystander. But the victim was okay and **threw** the ball back onto the field. Well, maybe not really "okay" but able to return the ball. She **rolled her legs and ankles around** to make sure nothing was broken. She **wiggled her toes**. She **put her heels and toes together**. Everything seemed to be okay with those extremities. She **made hammering movements** with her arms to make sure they were fine too. Other than a big bruise from being **knocked** down, she was okay. And thankful that it hit her and not her child. *(What might have been a preventative measure? Have you had an accident due to a sport?)*

The game continued with much **running** and **panting**. Tom **took a deep breath** and **closed his eyes**. He was remembering his youthful days again! Where had they gone so fast? The loud **cheering** of the crowd jerked him awake as he saw the ball sail quickly past the goalie. Unfortunately, it was not Justin's team!

Justin **looked down** at the ground and **pouted**. He was very tired and even **yawned**. He didn't like losing! Tom **got up** and gave his grandson a **hug**. He **smiled broadly** and said, "Let's get ice cream!" Justin **gave him a "high-five"** and **patted himself on the back**. Tom said, "Son, it's not about the winning, it's how you play the game. And how you handle losing says a lot about your character. Justin **waved** to the guys on the opposite team and **gave them a "thumbs up"**. *(What makes good sportsmanship? How do you handle losing?)*

"Great game", he said. "You really sneaked that last one by us…but we'll get you next time!" All the boys **nodded** and **laughed.**

"We'll see about that!" one of the others said and then they **laughed** again. Tom and Justin **licked** their cones vigorously. Justin was hungry and Tom was in a silly mood. He was thinking once again of his own childhood. Great memories! *(What great memories do you have from your childhood? What memories have you made with family? Is your family sports-oriented? Which sport? Do you know, or have you met, a famous sports figure?)*

Charlotte Saben, ADC, AP-BC

"Look up! **Look Up!**" Sadie **stretched** her neck and **rolled her head** as she gazed into the sky.

No one else saw anything unusual in the sky. (*What might you see in the sky? Have you ever seen anything unexpected...An UFO for example?*)

Jim **rolled his shoulders** in a shrug. "Nothing exciting up there!" he replied.

He continued to **move his shoulders forward and backward** and then **spread out his arms like an airplane.** "Vroom!" He **laughed** as he **made circles with his arms**. Then he **flapped his arms** and **cawed** like a bird. "I can fly! I can fly!" he mocked. (*Planes are designed after some characteristics of birds. Discuss this OR talk about birds in general...memories.*)

Sadie **bent over and touched her toes**. Anything to ignore that Jim! Perhaps if she **touched her knees AND toes**, he might think she was "addled" and go away!

Jim did, indeed **walk** away! In fact, he **marched** rather heavily out of the area!

Sadie's friend, Lily **sighed**. She **heaved her shoulders** and **took deep breaths** in and out. Jim always seemed to make fun of any situation. Lily had to **laugh**. And to admit that sometimes he was funny! (*Would you think Jim was funny? How would you respond?*)

But not this time. What was it that Sadie thought she saw? Lily wasn't sure she should ask. (*Have you ever been hesitant to ask a friend about something they said that you didn't understand? What did you do?*) So, she **made faces** hoping Sadie would **laugh**. Sadie **reached up and moved her arms in a swaying motion**. She **moved her feet in dancing steps.** She was listening to music in her head! Sadie had fun like that which was one reason Lily loved her. Perhaps Sadie had not seen anything in the sky. Perhaps she just wanted attention! (*Have you or someone you know done something silly or different just for attention? Tell us about it! Have you ever wanted to do something like that if you haven't?*)

(At this point you can play music and have them clap or use rhythm instruments, move their feet, etc.)

Sadie began to **clap**, and **stomp** her feet. She **rolled her ankles** and **tapped her toes**. She put her **heels together** and **then her toes** and made **swirling motions** with her hands. Sadie was obviously in another world!

Lily decided to join her. A few other people watching began *to point their fingers*, one at a time at the pair. No matter! They **lifted their legs one at a time** and **blinked their eyes** to the tune in their heads!

Jim returned and **looked up** to the sky. "Well, I'll be!" he said.

The ladies and the entire crowd gathered **looked up** too. And what to their wondering eyes should appear? (*YOU fill in the answer!*)

NOTE: If the residents need prompting, you can say…Santa Claus? A hot air balloon? A UFO?, etc.)

Charlotte Saben, ADC, AP-BC

He saw the lights **blinking** up ahead. Melvin was very curious about the commotion. It looked like the Police Station had **moved** to his street! He heard the loud sirens and **covered his ears**. He **made faces** of all kinds. Except for **smiling**. He wasn't going to do that until he found out what happened! (*What is something that would make you not want to smile? What sound might make you want to cover your ears?*)

His wife **slammed the screen door shut** in front of him. "Time to watch TV! Maybe there will be something on the news. That seems safer than **standing** there with the **door open**." She said. (*Have you ever been on the News? Did you ever witness something that was?*)

Melvin **looked to the left and then to the right**. He **looked up** as he saw the light from the helicopter. And then he **looked down** quickly and **shaded his face**. He **moved his arms wildly** like HE was a helicopter and Emily **pulled** with first her right and then her left arm to make him **step** back. He did **step back**, and then **forward** again! And then he **stepped to the side**!

The light pierced the evening sky and Melvin **walked** out onto the porch. He **bent down** to **pick up** a piece of paper, using **each finger to the thumb motion**. This mysterious note did not seem to want to be read! He finally got it! (*What do you think it said? Do you think Melvin should have stepped outside? What do you find hard to pick up with your fingers?*)

He **opened it** carefully because he didn't know where it had come from. Suddenly a policeman **ran up the steps** onto the porch!

"Give me that!" he demanded. Melvin should have obeyed the officer. But he didn't! He was too curious! He **held it high** above his head. Then he **opened one hand and then the other**. But the paper didn't fall down! Where did it go? (*Can you do any slight-of-hand tricks? Do you like magic? Do you think Melvin should obey the Officer? Would you?*)

Melvin knew the Officer was a patient man because he recognized him as his own son's best friend, Brian.

"You find that right now and give it to me!" The Officer was adamant. Melvin **laughed hard**. Then he produced the note by **reaching** into his pocket.

The Officer read the note and **made a puzzled face**. He **made several faces**!

"What?" he exclaimed.

Melvin **smiled** at the Officer. He got it! Now he understood exactly what was happening! He wasn't entirely sure the Officer did. *(How do you think Melvin knew?)*

Suddenly, a very bright light, not from the helicopter, encompassed Melvin. He did a little **dance**…he **touched his toes**. He **touched his heels together** and then **put his toes together**. He **smiled broadly** and **opened his arms wide**. He began to **sing**. *(What do you think he sang? Why? What is your favorite song to sing?)*

"What are you doing?" the Officer inquired.

"**Read** the noted again, Brian!" Melvin said as his son emerged, kicking a hat onto the porch. ***(Make motions like you are opening a note and reading it.)***

"Surprise!" he said.

Officer Brian looked stunned as the rest of the officers gathered around and began **clapping**. All this commotion was for…TV! Brian was secretly being filmed for a TV honorarium! He had won a national award!

Brian was stunned! Sll the lights, the **blinking**, the helicopter *(make blinking and helicopter motions again),* all the action…all to honor him!

Emily **opened the door** and **blew him a kiss**! She had his favorite cookies on a tray. "**Munch** away!" she said.

All of the officers, the actors, and the media began to **cheer** and **stomp** their feet. And, of course, **munch**! *(Have you ever seen a movie being made? Would you like to? Why or why not?) OR (What is your favorite cookie? Tell me what it smells like, feels like in your mouth!)*

Charlotte Saben, ADC, AP-BC

Colleen **walked** briskly into the kitchen. She smelled the coffee pot brewing and the cookies baking. She **took a deep breath in and out** and **shrugged her shoulder**s. She **rolled her neck around in circles** as this always helped her relax. Her girlfriends would be here soon. She had known several of them from way back in high school. She **kicked** at the dog dish on the floor and then **bent over** to **pick it up.** She **washed** her hands and **shook** them dry before **wiping** them on the towel. She **looked up** at the clock and then **down** at the floor. She should have time to **mop** if she got right on it. She **looked to the left and right** also. Where had she put that cookie plate? *(Do you have old friends from high school or college? Did you ever have a get-together with just girl (or guy) friends? What did you do?)*

Colleen loved having her friends over for craft night. Sometimes they **painted.** Sometimes they **knitted.** Sometimes they **cut and pasted**. She **reached up** in the cupboard and **pulled** out the cookie plate, because she suddenly remembered where it was. She **arranged** the cookies on it, **flipping them with quick wrist motion.** *(What hobbies did you have when you were younger? Which ones do you still enjoy? What is your favorite cookie? What ingredients do you think are in them? Do you like to bake?)*

She **stomped** her feet to scare the cat away from the hot oven door. "I swear that cat really does have nine lives and hasn't learned a thing from any of them!" she said out loud. The cat **leaped** across the counter and **pranced** out the door, **sticking her head and nose up** in the air arrogantly. Colleen **shook her head** and **laughed.** She **made faces** at the retreating animal. "Such a smug creature!" she thought to herself.

She got out the hammer and began to **pound** on the towel lying on the counter. Good thing that cat hadn't **knocked** that off. This was a newly discovered craft she wanted to present to her friends tonight. She **worked the dough** in the bowl, **kneading** it and **pressing** and **rolling** it. She hoped the girls would all like her plan. She knew they would like the cookies! *(What do you think she was pounding in the towel? Have you ever made something special with or for a friend?)*

The phone rang and she answered**, sitting** down in a chair. She **crisscrossed her legs** while chatting to Muriel, who was inquiring about tonight's craft. Muriel always had to know what to expect ahead of time, even if only a few minutes! Colleen tried to hang up the phone, but **dropped** it instead. **Reaching down** and **touching her toes**, she managed to retrieve the phone and place it in its cradle. She **made circles with her ankles** to alleviate the cramp she had. Then she **pushed** herself up with her hands on her knees. This helped **stretch** her aching back! *(Do you, or did you like talking on the phone to friends? What kind of exercise did you do?)*

Maureen, her next door neighbor, and part of the girlfriends craft group, **knocked** on the door. Colleen **opened** the door and **held it wide** for Maureen to bring the large basket of lemons inside. There might be time to make lemonade if she opted not to **mop** that floor! *(Would you have mopped or made lemonade? Why?)*

The evening went very well. They **glued** and **painted** and **chatted** and **ate** all at the same time. The shininess of their projects made them **smile**. The ladies were somewhat astonished at Colleen's new ideas. They loved her cookies as well. And the lemonade! *(What do you think the project might have been? What does it feel like to get glue on your hands? What about paint? What about chocolate? Tell me how you would get each of these off your hands?)*

Daniel **tossed** the potato into the air **and caught it** again. He did this several times before Mary noticed him. She **glared** at him and **shook her head**. She **looked to the right and then to the left**. It didn't appear that anyone else had seen him. THAT was good! She sometimes felt like she couldn't take Daniel anywhere! (*Have you had someone do something questionable in a store with you?*)

"Stop that!" Mary said it louder than she had meant to. Several people **looked up** at her. She **looked down**, trying to seem inconspicuous.

Daniel **threw** the potato back in the bin and **picked up** an orange. He **tucked** it under his arm and **reached** for another. Soon he was **juggling** three oranges. (*Do you know how to juggle? Would you like to try?*)

"Good job, Dan!" he said to himself. Mary **made faces** at him. She didn't want to attract attention to herself and especially not to him! She **walked** away from him, pretending not to know him. But he **ran** behind her, **juggling** all the way. He was proud of himself for being able to **walk and juggle** at the same time! He **put down** the oranges and **made a victory sign** behind Mary's head. (*What might that look like? Do you think it was a good thing or bad thing that he could juggle and walk at the same time…in the grocery store?*)

He **laughed**. He **raised his arms** and **made a fist and then displayed his muscles**. No one was **watching**. At least he didn't think so! He **opened and closed his hands** a few times. They get stiff easier than they used to. He didn't like that. (*Do you think someone may have been watching? What about cameras in the stores? How do you feel about that?*)

Mary **pushed t**he cart down the aisle. A bag of dishwashing bars had fallen open onto the floor. Mary **weaved** around them. Daniel **kicked** at them. They actually made great hockey pucks! He aimed for the stack of cleaning wipes on display.

"Stop it, Daniel!" Mary said it a little quieter this time. He **kicked** one more "puck" down the aisle. Great aim! It **shook** the display just enough to cause two cartons to fall onto the floor! Daniel **bent down** to pick everything up. He **touched his toes** and then **stood up** and did it all again!

"Daniel!" Mary's tone and volume was increasing. "This is no place to do your exercises! And it certainly isn't a hockey arena!" Daniel **smiled**.

"I'll go sit on the bench by the door." Daniel thought it would be safer and more entertaining than following Mary around! At least he could **look** at the other shoppers or perhaps **read** the ads. *(What things might he observe? Smell? See? Hear? Did you ever sit on a bench while others shopped?)*

"Can you stay out of trouble?" Mary wasn't sure she should take her eyes offm him. (***roll eyes around***)

Daniel **shrugged.** He **rolled his shoulders forward and backward** and **stretched his arms over his head**. He **swayed back and forth** for a few moments and then **stomped** off towards the bench.

He sat down and began to **make circles with his ankles**. Then he **moved his feet up and down and clicked his heels together and then his toes**. This was MUCH better than **wandering** down the aisles with Mary. *(What items might you have in your grocery cart? Did you have any aisles that you avoided? What is your favorite grocery store and why? And your favorite food from there?)*

Daniel noticed the clerks checking the customers through their lines. He started **moving his arms like he was scanning items** while **raising his eyebrows**. He was pretending to scan items on the conveyor belt. Silly Daniel! The clerks noticed Daniel and began to **laugh.** One started a little **dance, moving his shoulders and feet** to the beat of the scanner. This was fun!

By the time Mary arrived at the check-out line, all the clerks were **singing or humming and moving** to the "music" of a strange sound.

Yes! Daniel was **drumming** on his lap, **tapping his feet** and **singing at the top of his lungs!** And occasionally, he would lead the chorus by the **wave of his arms.** It caught on and the merriment seemed to make the whole day go faster for everyone!

But soon the store manager appeared, **scowling**. He **shook his finger** rapidly and then **pointed each one** at Daniel. And then **smiled broadly** and **recited his vowels**. He was just a strange as Daniel! Mary thought the manager might ask her not to bring Daniel again, but instead he scheduled him for "entertainment" on a regular weekly basis! They **shook hands** and **hugged.** *(Tellme about the funniest thing you ever saw while shopping. Share any shopping experience.)*

Charlotte Saben, ADC, AP-BC

Frankie **picked up** the cat and **stroked** its back. She **wiggled her fingers** and **opened and closed her hands** several times. This was THE big day! This was the day she had looked forward to for so long! The cat **jumped** off her lap as she **saluted** and **sat up straight**. She felt very proud! She **put both hands to her eyebrows and scoured the horizon**. He should be here any minute now. *(Have you ever been waiting for someone's arrival? Who? What did you feel?)*

She **gently kicked** at the cat which was playing with her untied shoelace. Then she **bent down** to **tie** her shoe. She didn't want her brother to meet her looking sloppy! After all, they had not been together in over 50 years! *(Have you ever been reunited with someone not seen for years?)*

Frankie **shook her head** at the memories that haunted her. She **rolled her neck around several times** trying to both forget and remember. *(What do you think might have happened?)*

They were just kids. They had been playing like they were birds **flying in** the air. She **spread out her arms and made both soaring and flapping motions** remembering how it felt. She **laughed.** She **rolled her ankles** the way her brother, Steve, had when he pretended to be a bird-helicopter! She **waved her arms above her head** in true helicopter fashion! Then she **swayed** them in the air like she had when "her" bird sat in the tree. She liked the **smell** of the pine trees in their mountain home. *(What smells do you remember? What is your favorite nature smell?)*

Her **smile faded** as she recalled the car **driving** up the dirt path to their place. In fact, she **made all kinds of faces**, releasing the painful memories. But she ended up **laughing** again at the silliness of it all. She is, after all, an adult now.

She **got up** and **walked** to the end of the porch. This time a car would be welcome! It would bring Steve back into her life! She did a little jig with her feet.

She practiced **waving her arms** in every possible way! She hoped Steve was still the funny, lovable guy she remembered. He just retired from the Navy. Maybe they could be a family again!

Steve, meanwhile, **stretched his whole body**, just waking from a dream. It had been a pleasant dream for the most part, partly of childhood with Frankie, and partly with adventures in the military. He **yawned**. Then he saw Frankie! His driver **beeped the horn** at his command.

Frankie **ran** to meet the automobile. Steve **opened the door** and **leaped** out. They gave each other the biggest of **hugs** ever! (***Hug yourself!***)

They had a LOT of catching up to do! Frankie's husband, Don, **poured** the coffee as they sat down to reminisce and reveal! They all **took a deep breath** and… *(What do you think they did next?)*

Charlotte Saben, ADC, AP-BC

Ruby loved the winter because she could **skate** outside on the pond instead of inside a building! *(Do you like winter? Do you live, or have you lived where people skate on the pond? Have you?)* She did a little **jig, bouncing her feet, toes up and then heels**, as she hunted for her skates. They were in the closet yesterday! She knew for sure because they had nearly **fallen** on her head when she **opened** it. ***(Besides the falling motions with hands and the opening motion, the residents could "duck" down as if avoiding an object from above, OR reach up as if holding it.)***

There they are! Ruby **bent down** and **pulled** her skates on. She **laced** them quickly **moving her fingers agilely**. She **touched her toes** and **used her hands on her knees to push herself up again**. She loved skating. She **lifted her arms** in the air and **swayed**. She **moved them in circles** just imagining herself in the Olympics! She **made figure eights with her arms, fingers entwined**. Then she **made them with her legs!** *(Have you ever been in or desired to be in the Olympics? Some other sporting challenge? What other dream have you had? What would it feel like to be skating in an outdoor pond? Do you think there is a difference in feeling between a pond and an indoor rink? Why or why not? What differences?)*

Brad came around the corner and **peeked** in through Ruby's door. "Silly girl!" he said. "Ice skating like that is silly! It's not a sport! It's sissy stuff!"

"It is not!" Ruby retorted immediately. "And get out of my room! I don't even want your eyes in my room!" Brad **rolled his eyes** at her and **moved his head from left to right and up and down.**

"No one here to verify my presence", he said matter-of-factly. The he **knocked** on her door faster and faster. He **rolled his wrists in circles** as if leading a band and began to **march in place**. He did this just to irritate his sister. *(Did you and a sibling do things just to bug each other? How about your children? Grandchildren?)*

"The ONLY **skating** that is worth it is hockey! He **swung his arms** wildly as if making a goal. He **raised his arms in the air** and **made a fist and then a V for victory** with his fingers. "That's where REAL skaters play!"

Ruby **took off her skates** and **flung** them over her shoulders. She **walked** past Brad, **giving him a little shove.** *(Do you like hockey better than figure skating?)*

"Humph!" she said. He **made a face** at her. She **ran** out the door and down the street to the pond.

There was a group of boys practicing hockey at one end of the pond. "Silly boys!" she thought. "Always have to feel macho!" *(Make muscles with arms.)* She **bent** again to put on her skates. But this time she did not touch her toes. She **wiggled** them instead and **moved her ankles in circles**.

She **glided** out onto the ice far away from the boys. She **made graceful motions** with both arms and legs. She felt the cold air against her cheeks and **moved her mouth around** so her lips wouldn't freeze. She **patted her cheeks.** She **patted her back.** She **rubbed her thighs.** It was colder than she had thought! "BRRR" she said. After only a short time, she **stepped** off the ice and removed her skates. Even the boys had put away their sticks and were **stomping** the snow from their heads. Ruby **shook her head** and **moved it slowly around in circles**. She preferred to watch the snow from her window. Skating while snowing was not usually a good idea for her. She wasn't known as "Grace" on the ice. She might **slip**.

She turned her feet inward with her toes touching. This unfroze her ankles. She **jogged** to the house just as the snow began to fall rapidly. *(Make motions like the snow is falling with fingers and arms.)*

She **laughed** at the sight of Brad **shoveling** snow on the patio. Dad must be home! And, she **heaved her shoulders** in laughter at remembering that her parents had just installed a camera in the hallway! What a good day it had been! *(Why would a camera be funny? What does she think they might have discovered? OR Have you ever had to shovel snow? Run a snowplow? Got caught in a blizzard? Describe the feel and sounds of a blizzard.)*

Charlotte Saben, ADC, AP-BC

Big Tim **pulled** his pistol out of his pocket and **twirled** it around his fingers. He was pretty good at that. In fact, he held the record for the fastest pistol spinner in the west. *(Can you spin a gun or object on your fingers? Do you like western shows?)*

Little Claude was about to change that. He **marched** up to the saloon and **flung** open the doors. "Put 'em up, Tim!" he yelled. Claude refused to use the terms "big" or "little". He didn't think they mattered. What mattered was what he held in his hand! "You're goin' down, Bro!" he taunted. (***Make faces or show "power sign"!)***

Big Tim **heaved his shoulders** and **laughed** heartily. "Right!" he said. "And I s'pose YOU'RE the one gonna do it?" Tim **threw** his water bottle across the counter. "Ok. I'll put 'em up just for you!" He **laid** his pistol on the counter and **made a fist** with his hands. He **opened his fist**. He did this several times. Then he **moved his fingers independently** as if trying to figure which one to use to **pull** the trigger. He **made a face**. He **made a mean face**. He **made a silly face**. He **licked his chops**. And then he **smiled broadly**. He **picked up** his pistol. The men in the saloon **cheered**. The ladies did a few **dance steps**, but rather cautiously. There was a lot of chatter. (***Make motions like people are talking either with mouth or fingers.*** *(How do you feel when someone challenges you?)*

Just then Little Claude **dropped** something on the floor. The place went silent. SHHH! (***Make quiet sign with finger to lips.)*** He **bent down** to **pick it up**. He **touched the toes** of his boots and **then his knees**, and then **slid** the items across the floor. Those who saw it **gasped**! *(would you have been startled by it? What would startle you?)*

Was this a challenge to the death? One of the spectators began to **cry** and then **giggled.** Another **lifted** his glass in the air and **waved** it around. He **stared** at the object on the floor and then **jumped** as it **scampered** past. *(Would you feel scared if you were in this saloon at this moment? Why or why not?)*

Little Claude **swung** his pistol around and **pointed** it at Big Tim. Big Tim **drew** his, **swinging his arms up and around** in gigantic gestures. The people in the line of fire **ducked, moving their heads up and down and to the left and right.** Where was that sheriff when you needed him? They also **kicked** at the tables as they hid under them! Some of them **folded their hands to pray.**

Suddenly Lady Donna **pushed** the doors wide and **pranced** up to the bar. She **dropped** towels on the heads of those patrons who did not make it under the tables! *(Could they be crying towels? What is a crying towel?)*

"On yer mark!" she yelled. "Get set! SHOOT!" She **made circles with her arms** as she almost as if she were trying **point** them in a different direction.

Tim and Claude **squeezed** their triggers! But instead of a "Bang!" out came_____ *(You decide: water as in squirt guns? Silly string? Paint balls? Air? What kinds of pistols or guns have you seen?)*

Then someone in the crowd started **stomping**. "Get that thing away from me!" they screamed. *(What thing were they talking about?)*

Everyone started **laughing** and **slapping their knees**. "Look at Big Tim! I think he lost this duel!" Tim looked dejectedly at his pistol which was **dripping** with cool-aide! He **wiped** his face with his sleeve. The trigger was dripping with sugar and Tim's hands were a sticky mess. He **shook** his wrists and **wiggled his fingers**. *(What kind of Kool-Aide do you like? How about snow cones? What kind of sticky mess have you been in? What did it look, taste, smell, feel, and sound like?)*

"Who put THAT stuff in there?" Tim demanded to know. Just then the object on the floor **reached** his foot. Tim **shook his ankle** trying to get it off. The crowd roared with laughter! Tim had indeed lost this battle of the squirt guns! And the remote-controlled cockroach had done him in indeed! Everyone **clapped** and had a great time! And no one died…only the batteries on the remote bug! *(Do you think they thought the bug was real when Claude first dropped it on the floor? Who was controlling the cockroach? Have you ever touched a cockroach? What did it feel like? What feeling do you get when you see a real one?)*

     Charlotte Saben, ADC, AP-BC

Julia saw it first! "It's a coyote!" she declared.

"No, it's only a dog…a very lonely and scruffy dog" replied Joe, as he **stepped out of the car.** *(Have you ever seen a strange stray animal? Did you ever see an animal that you were not sure what it was? What is the scariest animal you ever encountered face to face?)*

Julia was more cautious as she **tiptoed** across the lot so as not to disturb the animal. She **glared** at Joe. She wasn't sure he was right and that animal was only a few feet away. She decided she would **run** instead and take her chances on the beast chasing her. Joe was not so nimble and sort of **marched** rather heavily but quickly behind her. Finally, they slowed their pace to a more normal **walking** speed, but Joe was **crisscrossing** his legs to be silly because he was nervous. *(Why was he nervous? What makes you nervous?)*

They **opened** the door to the restaurant and **looked** around. Julia **moved her head to the right and to the left** looking for a cozy booth. Joe **looked up** at the ceiling, hoping for a spot away from the fans. His eyes caught the menu posted above and he **rolled his eyes**. He **rolled** his neck! Then he **reached** into his pocket. *(What would you find in your pocket or purse? What is the most unusual thing you have had there?)* When he **pulled** out his hand, he **opened** and **closed** it, and out fell a quarter! He **bent over** to **pick** it up. He had a hard time getting it, and tried with **each of his fingers pressed to the thumb…on both hands!** Finally, the waitress retrieved it for him and led them to their seats. They **walked** softly to the booth and **sat, stretching their legs**. "Did you see that coyote out there?" Julia asked the waitress.

"It's just a stray dog," corrected Joe.

"Yes, he hangs out here a lot. Gets into the garbage once in a while. Animal control can't seem to **catch** him. Not sure what it is."

Joe **sipped** at his water as he looked at the menu. He **puckered** when his lips touched the lemon wedge. He forgot to say "No lemon, please".

Julia **tossed** her salad vigorously. The restaurants never do it right in her opinion. Joe **stirred** his soup. He **crunched** the crackers into it with **his fingers**. Then they both **squeezed** the honey into their tea.

"You do know it's a coyote, don't you Joe?" Julia asked.

"Nope! It's a dog! A scroungy mutt, I'd say."

Julia **made a face** at Joe. She even **stuck out her tongue!** Joe was wrong but he wouldn't admit it. She pretended to tell him off by **accentuating her vowels** but quietly, almost under her breath.   This relieved her tension.   She **rolled her shoulders** forward and then backwards. It made her relax a bit. If only Joe wouldn't be so stubborn! (*How do you feel when you think you are right and someone else is wrong? What do you do?*) She **reached** out her arms in a playful **punching** manner. She **jabbed** at Joe across the table. But she didn't hit him. She only envisioned **socking** him in the nose! She **laughed** out loud at the thought. She would never really do that! Maybe that critter is a dog…

Joe **stretched his arms over his head** as if lifting a weight. He **stretched to the right and then the left** and put up his playful dukes too. He made a **jabbing motion with his elbows** as if Julia were seated beside him instead of across the table. He didn't know why he did that, just for fun.

The waitress interrupted the duel with the main dishes they had ordered. They began to **eat rapidly** as if in a competition. *(What do like to order from a restaurant? Do you eat fast or slowly?)*

When they finished, and paid the bill, they both **waved** their arms to say goodbye. They **opened** the door to see the animal waiting by their car! Joe **threw** his leftover's bag at the beast who promptly **gobbled** it up and **ran** into the field.

Joe **laughed** as he admitted "Maybe that was a coyote after all!" Julia pretended to **kick** at him, **laughing** nervously at the thought of the animal almost getting a ride with them! *(Have you ever had a "wild" animal for a pet?" What is the most unusual pet you have had? What did you name it? Did Joe and Julia use good manners in the restaurant? Why do you think that way? What would a coyote look like? What might it sound, feel like?)*

Then they **smiled** and **hugged**. And even **blew kisses**.

Charlotte Saben, ADC, AP-BC

Jane **loved** *(hugging self)* going to the pet store. She often **walked** there with her friend. Her friend **wheeled** her wheelchair over the curb and **looked up** at the closed door. She **looked to the right and to the left** but saw no one. She wasn't sure Jane could **lift** her over the door jamb and **open the door** at the same time. Jane **laughed** at her. "I am woman!" She said. "I can do this!" She **raised her arms** and **made a power sign**. *(What makes you feel powerful?)*

Just then a young man **ran** up to them. He **pulled** the door open and **yelled** for a clerk to **hold** it. He **squeezed** his hands around the handles of the wheelchair. With just one **push** she was over the hump and in the store.

"Thank you so much!" She said.

"No problem," the young man replied. "I like to help when I can. He **bent down** to give her **a hug**. "Thank you for the opportunity!" She **patted him on the back**.

"What a nice young man! You certainly don't find them everywhere anymore!" Jane said. She started to comment further when she realized a cute puppy was **pawing** at the window, **begging** to be held. *(How do animals beg? Let's see some begging eyes! Did you give in to your pet's begging?)* She **stroked** the puppy. She **moved her fingers through his fur**. He **licked** her face. *(I don't suggest actually licking, but the tongue motion alone)* She smiled broadly. Then she **reached** down and let the puppy **touch her toes**. She **wiggled her toes** and **shook her ankles** while the puppy tugged at her shoes. She **made circles with her feet** while he chased them.

After the puppy tired, which didn't take too long, she **reached out** and took a cat into her lap. She **played pat-a-cake** with the cat on her lap. She **clapped her hands** in delight which startled the cat which then **leaped** off her lap and **scampered** away. *(What noises startle you? Tell me about a cat you had. Are you allergic to any animals?)*

Jane **reached out with her arms** to try to catch the cat, but it was already hiding in the shelves. So, she **hugged** herself instead! Then she **danced** her way over to the birds where a cockatiel lit on her shoulder. She **rolled her shoulders** to see if he would fly off. But he didn't! She **rolled her neck both ways**, and still he **strutted** on her shoulder! He **stared** at her. She **rolled her eyes** and **made faces**. Still he perched! Finally, she **stuck out her arms**

and made circles and movements as if **flying** herself! And then she tried to **make bird calls!**

That did it! No proper bird was going to sit around and listen to that nonsense! He **hopped** back into his cage! He told her off in no uncertain terms in the real bird language! *(Did you ever own a talking bird? Train a bird? If you were a bird, what kind, color, would you like to be? What would you sound like? Eat? Etc. Have you ever tried communicating with any animal?)*

She **looked down** and saw some turtles **splashing** in the tub on the floor. They looked much calmer than any of the other pets she had experienced so far that day! But she knew that she did not want to change their habitat frequently, so they did not appeal to her as pets. *(Did you ever have an aquarium? Do you like fish? To eat? To have as pets?)*

The one pet that she did enjoy was the fish! She liked watching them **swim** and **twist** through the aquarium's rocks and bridges. And they didn't need as frequent care! Just the **dropping** in a few pebbles of food daily. A snail would take care of a lot of the cleaning. *(**Make a dropping and then wiping or cleaning motion.**)*

But Jane enjoyed the animals best when they were at the pet store and not in her care! So, she found her friend, who was surrounded *(**make huge circles with arms in the front as if encompassing everyone**)* by the store staff trying to rescue her from their one and only monkey! He was **swinging his arms** and **kicking** the wall and in general making a scene! *(Have you ever been involved with a monkey? How are they like humans? How are they different? Would you be afraid of a monkey? Why? Why not? What animal might you be afraid of?)*

Jane and her friend made it home safely. They **zigzagged** across the street and **smiled** at everyone they say. They had a wonderful adventure! Now they would settle down and **listen to music** and **eat** their dinner. They would leave the animals to the handlers! *(What is your favorite type of music? Food?)*

Charlotte Saben, ADC, AP-BC

"Howdy!" Randy **shouted** to the crowd. It wasn't his first rodeo and he knew what he was doing and what he wanted! *(What does the phrase "not his first rodeo" mean? Have you ever been to a rodeo? Where was it?)*

He **rode** his horse up to the fence where he **scanned** the audience. *(make motion like you are searching the audience…hand cupped to eye, etc.)* He was looking for his cousin, Ned, so he could show him how to **rope** a calf! It wasn't the **twirling the rope** that bothered Ned, but the **tying up** of the calf. *(Do you think this practice is okay? Why or why not? Do you like rodeos?)*

Justine, Randy's girlfriend **galloped** up to join him. She preferred **barrel racing** to roping any day. *(Make figure eights with legs or arms to indicate the barrel racing.)* And she was the champ! She **held** her trophy **high above her head**. She **waved** it in the air and **made "thumbs up" signs** with her hands. Randy **pointed to her with outstretched arm** and began to **clap** his hands. The audience responded with vigorous **clapping** and even **stomping their feet**!

Ned **climbed** down from the bleachers and walked to the fence. He knew what Randy wanted. He **made a sad face**. He **made a mad face**. He **shook his fist** at Randy and then he **marched** away. *(Why was Ned angry? Did you ever do something for your family that you didn't really want to do?)*

Randy **spurred** his horse gently. For some reason the horse **reared**, nearly **knocking** Randy off! "Hey, Buddy!" Randy said. "It's okay. Ned wasn't really that angry!" Randy **looked to the right and then to the left** but couldn't see Ned anywhere! "He probably went somewhere to **pout**!" Randy said aloud.

Meanwhile Justine was **waving her arms in circles** trying to get the attention of the clowns. They would need to be ready for the next event…the bull riders! *(Do you like clowns? Tell me about a happy or sad experience with clowns. Do you think they are good for rodeos? Circuses? Children's parties? Why or why not?)*

Bull riders have to be tough! They **bounce** in the saddle and **hang** on for dear life! But the clowns must be brave! They get the bulls to **chase** them. The clowns came out and **ran** around the arena. They **smiled** at the crowd. Then they **pulled** out their red flags and began to practice teasing the bulls. *(Make waving motions from side to side as if holding a red flag)*

Suddenly the **whistle blew**! Randy and Justine **snapped** the reins and exited the arena.

Tom **climbed** onto Big Henry, the most challenging bull! The gate **opened**. The crowd **gasped**. Then several **breathed in and out** trying to relax! Who would win? Big Henry was very good at **tossing** off cowboys!

One clown **bent** down to tie his shoe just as the gate **swung** wide! *(Do you think the bull charged him? Do you think Tom stayed on or fell off?)*

He **dropped** a ball out of his pocket. He needed that for his magic trick! So he tried to **pick it up with his fingers**. He **pinched** each of them against the ball, but it kept **rolling** closer and closer to Big Henry! Yikes!

The crowd **looked up**! Something was **sailing** through the air! Not something… someone! *(Was it Tom the cowboy or the clown or something else?)* Big Henry had won again in one way or another.

Randy **kicked** at the dirt and moved his feet with a **toe tapping** motion. He **rolled his ankles** trying to decide what to do. He really did see Ned's point, but he was a COWBOY! And the calves did not get hurt! In fact, they seemed to **prance** around after the roping, in his opinion. *(What does a rodeo smell like? What might you eat at a rodeo? Hear? Would you like to be a cowboy? Have you ever ridden a horse? Do you think the horse liked to be ridden?)*

Ned came **strolling** over to Randy, **crisscrossing his legs** in a drunken style even though he had not been **drinking.** "Let's just agree to disagree on this, okay?" he asked.

"Whatever," said Randy. "I just want your support." *(How can you give support to someone if you disagree with them?)*

"Of course!" Ned said. "I support your being a cowboy because that is who you are! And you're a darn good one too! Besides, I LOVE horses and you give me opportunities to **watch** them in action!" He **gave his cousin a hug** and **waved** goodbye. They would always be good friends. And Ned may never reveal that secretly he would like to be a cowboy too! *(Did you have friends or relatives who are very different from you?) (Tell us about what you did for a career when you were younger.) (Share a dream or secret desire you may have had.)*

Charlotte Saben, ADC, AP-BC

Mark **pulled** his hat on his head and then **shook his head**. He **looked to the left and then the right**, slower this time. **He looked up.** Yeah, it looks like possible **rain.** Not today, please. He **looked up** again **and then down**. How could it threaten to rain when he had a day off to go **fishing**? *(Would you go fishing on a rainy day? Why or why not?)*

He wasn't sure whether he should **call** Sam and cancel or risk it anyway. If it didn't produce **lightning**, they would be okay in a storm. He **swayed back and forth, waving his arms in the air.** If the trees can handle a little **wind and rain**, why can't men? He **made a fist** with his hand and **displayed his muscles**. He **opened and closed his hands.** His arthritis seems to be under control, so the storm can't be too bad. Maybe it won't hit at all! *(Does your body give signs of weather changes?)*

Sam was right on time, as usual. He **drove** up rapidly and **screeched the brakes**. He **moved his feet up and down** as he **turned off** the engine. He **made circular motions with his ankles**. Yep! His arthritis told him the storm might indeed hit! He didn't care! He'd been out in much worse weather! He recalled **running** to the cellar as a kid, trying to avoid the tornado that threatened his community. He had **jumped i**nto the cellar just in time. The tornado passed through without **touching** down. Whew! *(Have you ever lived in tornado country? Had to hide in a basement or cellar?)*

And then there was the time when he went **bicycling** in the rain. He had to **swerve** the handlebars to keep upright. Even then, he made a lot of **splashing**. The thunder startled him and he **pedaled faster**. He had **made faces** up towards Heaven because his dad had told him thunder was God's **bowling** team and lightning was the angels **taking pictures**. They could get a good one for him that day, but it wasn't a **smile!** *(What stories were you told as a child to explain things of nature? Did you ever ride a bicycle in the rain?)*

Sam **walked** over to Mark and **stuck out his hand for a shake**. Then he **patted** him on the back.

"Ready to go?" he asked.

"Think we ought to?" Mark answered with another question.

"But of course! The rain ain't never stopped me before, and it ain't gonna start at my age!" Sam was determined to go fishing.

The men **dragged** their gear to Mark's pick up and **threw i**t in the truck bed. Sam **dropped** a container of worms and **bent** over to retrieve as many as possible. Some of them **slithered** away and attracted several birds. They began **flapping** and **cawing** loudly. The men **covered their ears** and shooed the birds away by **clapping** their hands. *(What kinds of gear to you think they brought? What would you have taken? What kinds of birds would you see? What would they look and sound like?)*

The **drive** there wasn't bad. Once the boat was in the water, the men **rowed** away from the shore. Because they were long-time buddies and no one else was around, they began to **sing** silly songs. Sometimes this was more fun than **fishing.** *(Do you have a long-time friend? What fun things did you do with them? What silly song comes to mind in this story? Let's sing a few lines.)*

Eventually they settled down and **cast their lines** into the quiet water. Sam almost fell asleep and began to **snore** slightly. He had barely **rolled his neck** to wake himself up when he suddenly felt a **pull** on his line, which was secured between his knees. He **reeled** it in slowly. A BIG catfish! That will make a great supper! The wind had **kicked** up and rain came down in buckets. The adventure would have to end. At least they had a catfish! Well, Sam did! Mark **threw** out his line one final time and **reeled** it in again. Someone Above was **smiling** on him, because on the end of his hook was a small bass. Yes, smaller, but still good eating! And enough …just enough for dinner. *(Do you like to fish? What kinds of fish have you caught? What kind do you like best to eat? What do you eat with fish? Describe the smell, feel, taste, etc.)*

What a happy day! Both men **breathed in and out deeply** several times once they were safely on the road home…happy campers…er, fishermen and friends!

Charlotte Saben, ADC, AP-BC

Colleen **walked** briskly into the kitchen. She smelled the coffee pot brewing and the cookies baking. She **took a deep breath in and out** and **shrugged her shoulder**s. She **rolled her neck around in circles** as this always helped her relax. Her girlfriends would be here soon. She had known several of them from way back in high school. She **kicked** at the dog dish on the floor and then **bent over** to **pick it up.** She **washed** her hands and **shook** them dry before **wiping** them on the towel. She **looked up** at the clock and then **down** at the floor. She should have time to **mop** if she got right on it. She **looked to the left and right** also. Where had she put that cookie plate? *(Do you have old friends from high school or college? Did you ever have a get-together with just girl (or guy) friends? What did you do?)*

Colleen loved having her friends over for craft night. Sometimes they **painted.** Sometimes they **knitted.** Sometimes they **cut and pasted**. She **reached up** in the cupboard and **pulled** out the cookie plate, because she suddenly remembered where it was. She **arranged** the cookies on it, **flipping them with quick wrist motion.** *(What hobbies did you have when you were younger? Which ones do you still enjoy? What is your favorite cookie? What ingredients do you think are in them? Do you like to bake?)*

She **stomped** her feet to scare the cat away from the hot oven door. "I swear that cat really does have nine lives and hasn't learned a thing from any of them!" she said out loud. The cat **leaped** across the counter and **pranced** out the door, **sticking her head and nose up** in the air arrogantly. Colleen **shook her head** and **laughed.** She **made faces** at the retreating animal. "Such a smug creature!" she thought to herself.

She got out the hammer and began to **pound** on the towel lying on the counter. Good thing that cat hadn't **knocked** that off. This was a newly discovered craft she wanted to present to her friends tonight. She **worked the dough** in the bowl, **kneading** it and **pressing** and **rolling** it. She hoped the girls would all like her plan. She knew they would like the cookies! *(What do you think she was pounding in the towel? Have you ever made something special with or for a friend?)*

The phone rang and she answered**, sitting** down in a chair. She **crisscrossed her legs** while chatting to Muriel, who was inquiring about tonight's craft. Muriel always had to know what to expect ahead of time, even if only a few minutes! Colleen tried to hang up the phone, but **dropped** it instead. **Reaching down** and **touching her toes**, she managed to retrieve the phone and place it in its cradle. She **made circles with her ankles** to alleviate the cramp she had. Then she **pushed** herself up with her hands on her knees. This helped **stretch** her aching back! *(Do you, or did you like talking on the phone to friends? What kind of exercise did you do?)*

Maureen, her next-door neighbor and part of the girlfriends' craft group, **knocked** on the door. Colleen **opened** the door and **held it wide** for Maureen to bring the large basket of lemons inside. There might be time to make lemonade if she opted not to **mop** that floor! *(Would you have mopped or made lemonade? Why?)*

The evening went very well. They **glued** and **painted** and **chatted** and **ate** all at the same time. The shininess of their projects made them **smile**. The ladies were somewhat astonished at Colleen's new ideas. They loved her cookies as well. And the lemonade! *(What do you think the project might have been? What does it feel like to get glue on your hands? What about paint? What about chocolate? Tell me how you would get each of these off your hands?)*

George **walked** into the stadium, **stepping high** over the curb. He **reached** into his pocket and **pulled out** his ticket. As he **flung** it to the attendant, he **waved** at the bus driver who had brought him safely there. George liked the way Molly **drove** the bus. He secretly thought she was kind of cute too. *(Who will tell us about a time when you had a crush on someone? Your first kiss?)*

He **turned to the side**, **moving his head to the right and then to the left**. He was sure Dan and Clara would be here today! He **looked up**. No clouds. Dan hated cloudy days! *(What would you see right now if you looked up? What is the strangest thing you have ever seen by looking up? OR do you like cloudy days? What does a cloudy day make you feel like?)*

He **looked down**. Good thing too! The boy in front of him **threw** a snow cone onto the sidewalk! He **stepped over** it. He **stepped around** it. IN fact, he did a little **two-step slide** while onlookers **laughed.** George was somewhat of a show-off!

He found his seat after **looking** hard and **squinting** his eyes to see. He **sat** down. *(If residents are already seated or in wheelchairs, they can pat their laps to this remark. They can also put their hand up over their brows as if looking for something.)* He **slapped his knees** to the beat of the background music. He **made a fist and then released** it. He did this several times. He thought it would prepare his fingers for gestures he might make at the umpires. Hopefully, it will only be a **shaking fist**. He **shook his hands vigorously.**

He did not find Dan and Clara. George enthusiastically **started "the wave"** in the stadium. He loved seeing so many people exercise! He **swung his arms** as if he was the batter and **yelled** "Good eye!" when the pitch was called a ball. *(What other terms are used in a baseball game? Did you ever play baseball? Did you ever coach a team?)*

George loved everything that went with baseball. He **tipped his head up** to drink his beer (or soda) and guzzled it down. He **munched** on the nachos and **opened wide** to engulf the hot dog! *(What is your favorite thing to munch on? What does that smell like? Describe the taste and texture.)*

At the Seventh Inning Stretch, he **marched** quickly to the men's room. He **washed his hands** and **dried them on his pants**. He **stood straight** as he **sang**, rather exuberantly, "Take Me Out to the Ball Game!" He **reached** into his pocket and **waved** a five-dollar bill at the barker carrying popcorn. The bill dropped to the floor. George **bent down** to **pick it up**. His fingers couldn't quite **grasp** the bill. He **moved his fingers separately pushing**

them off his thumbs. Suddenly he got the bill between his index and thumb. YAY! *(Show me which your index finger is. Do you have trouble grasping things? What do you do?)*

He **stood up straight** again, but missed the vendor! Oh well! He had peanuts in his pocket anyway! He **licked his lips** at the thought. He **smacked** them loudly too, as he **sat** down!

"What!? What just happened?! Are you blind?" George was back focused on the game and not very happy with the umpire. He **made several faces**!

And then it happened! The moment George had been hoping for all his life! A foul ball was heading his way! But he didn't have a glove! Should he try to **catch** it bare-handed? *(Would YOU?)* He didn't have to think long about it as the ball **bounced** off the awning and right into his lap!

"Ouch and Hallelujah!" George declared. The burning of his lap was not so bad. He got the ball! And to make things even better, his favorite batter had hit it…just to him! *(Share experiences about being at a ball game.) (Share about your favorite team.)*

When the video monitor **zoomed** in on him, George **smiled broadly** and **waved wildly, holding up** his ball. As it scanned the audience, he spotted Dan and Clara…sitting right up front! He would have to find out how they finagled that!

As he exited the stadium, he **cradled** the ball, almost **hugging himself** in the process. He **jogged** a bit and **took large steps** as he boarded the bus. He **winked** at Molly, who winked back. Hey! George had had quite a day!

Charlotte Saben, ADC, AP-BC

Eric loved birds. He liked to take his binoculars and watch them in the early morning. ***(make circle shapes around the eyes like binoculars and move head from side to side)***. He liked the wake-up calls they made. *(Can you make bird calls? How did you wake up your family?)*

Sometimes, when no one was watching, Eric would **flap his arms** like he could fly. He knew he couldn't, but it was fun to pretend, even at his age. He sometimes **made circular motions with his arms**, starting with **small circles and getter bigger!** He thought this would increase his "flappability!" He knew if his daughter saw him that she would think he was nutty. He **made a face** at the thought. She kept too close of an eye on him, in his own opinion! He **moved his head to the left and then to the right**. He **looked down**. He **looked up**.

That's when he saw it! The very bird he had been trying to track. His favorite bird in the whole world. He **tiptoed** behind the bush. He **reached up** to **pull** away the leaves on the branch of the bush blocking his view. He **swayed** back and forth, trying to regain his balance. He **kicked** at a rock in the way. Then he **high-stepped** a few feet closer. Eric **tripped** a bit, and **dropped** his binoculars.

"Darn!" he said as he **bent** down to retrieve them. He **squatted**, half-way down, and **pushed himself up with his hands on his knees**. *(You can use a leaning motion with hands on knees and then a pushing up motion into an upright sitting position if your residents are in wheelchairs or sitting.)* The he decided to **touch his toes** several times since the precious bird had already taken **flight**. Might as well make this a useful event! He **touched his knees too and came to an upright position**. *(See above comment.)* He saw a log next to the bush and **sat** down on it. He **made circles with his feet** because he'd felt a little twinge when he **walked** to the log. He hoped the **movement** would alleviate the situation. *(Do you like morning exercise? What makes you twinge? How do you alleviate it? Share about any home remedies you tried.)*

He **moved his fingers, each individually to the thumb**. He **made wrist circles** like he was tossing a salad. It was still a beautiful morning. **He opened and closed his hands several times** around the binoculars. Fortunately, they were not scratched!

He felt very lucky! He had, indeed seen the special bird, even if not as close he wished. AND his binoculars survived the fall. He **rolled his neck in both directions** and **closed his eyes** briefly. He **took several deep breaths**. He **blinked** and then **sat up straight**! He

rolled his shoulders to make sure he was wide awake. There was his special bird again, not more than two feet away, looking straight at him! He wondered if the bird knew how much he loved him. He **whistled** quietly. He **puckered his lips** and **blew the bird a kiss**. The bird did not **fly** away! Eric **sat very still**. He **rolled his eyes** a bit to make sure he examined every part of the bird.

The bird accommodated him by **turning slowly** without taking flight. *(**If your residents are wheelchair bound or unable to turn, have them move from side to side as far as they can.**)* *(Have you ever made a special connection with an animal? What did it feel like? What is your favorite animal and why?)*

Eric was exuberant! His day had started off wonderfully. The bird seemed to sense that Eric had enough excitement for the day and **flew** off. Eric **waved** goodbye. He **did a little jig** and **clicked his heels together**. *(What would make you that excited?)*

He heard his daughter **calling**. No use trying to pretend he didn't. She would just come **running** down the path **scowling** and worried. She couldn't understand his being outside this early. *(What is your favorite time of day and why?)*

"I'm coming, Darlin'!" he said. Nothing could spoil his day now. Not even having to **eat** oatmeal for the fourth day in a row! His daughter isn't a morning person. Breakfast is boring! She will never understand. Eric **smiled broadly** and **marched** back into the house. He **hugged** his daughter and **gave himself a slap on the back!** He had already had a fantastic day while his daughter was **sleeping!** *(What is your favorite breakfast food? What does it smell, taste, and feel like? How do you prepare it?) OR (What common likes do you share with your children? How are you different? How do feel about your differences?)*

Charlotte Saben, ADC, AP-BC

Martha wasn't entirely sure what Fred's intentions were, but she really didn't care too much either. She **shook her head from side to side** and **heaved** a big sigh. She **scratched her head** and **rolled her neck around**. Why was it that she so looked forward to these Bingo Night Dates? Well, she probably shouldn't call it a "date" although she wouldn't mind if Fred thought of it as such. She did a little **jig** with her feet. She **patted** her heart which had begun to **flutter.** *(Do you remember your first crush? Who was the first to make your heart flutter? How old were you?)*

Fred **knocked** rather loudly on the door. He preferred the hardy **rap** to a simple **push** of the doorbell. It made him feel manly! He **shook his hands** afterwards and **rolled his wrists in circles**. Darned arthritis! He **opened and closed his hands** several times preparing for another **knock.** *(What makes you feel manly or womanly?)*

Martha **walked** to the door quickly and then **slowed** to a more "proper" pace. She didn't want to seem too enthusiastic! That would not be lady-like! *(What mannerisms do think "ladies" or "gentlemen" should do?)*

She **opened** it slowly and pretended to be surprised. "Oh, My! Is it Bingo night again, Fred? Why, you just come on in and I'll go get ready!"

Fred **smiled.** "You look mighty nice just the way you are!" He **winked** teasingly at her. She **rolled her eyes** and **scampered** off to the bathroom. *(Do you think she was already ready? What does a lady do to get ready for a date?)*

Martha **brushed her hair and teeth**. She **sprayed** on her favorite perfume…not too much…but just enough! She **tapped her feet** to make sure her shoes fit properly. She didn't want any clothing malfunctions tonight! *(What is your favorite perfume/cologne? Have you ever had a "wardrobe malfunction'?)*

Fred **side-stepped** the cat, Carlos, who **rubbed** up against his leg. He wouldn't **kick** him away, but he did **clap his hands** to shoo him off. Fred liked cats okay, but his nose didn't! He **made a face** to keep from sneezing. **He made several faces** before Martha **marched** back into the room. *(Do you like cats? Are you allergic to any animals?)*

"Is Carlos bothering you? That cat usually hates strangers." Martha said.

"Who are you calling a stranger? I'm not <u>that</u> strange! And he's seen me before!" Fred replied. "And besides, what's to hate about me? *(What is the strangest, most unique thing about you?)*

Martha wanted to say "Absolutely nothing!" but she didn't. Instead she **reached** for her shawl and purse. She **dropped** her glasses and **bent down** to retrieve them. Carlos **leaped** right in front of her causing her to **sway** back and forth for a moment. She **stretched her arms out** to regain her balance as Fred **reached** to assist her. Their hands met! Martha **blushed. *(Fan faces with hands as if embarrassed or hot.)*** Then she **pulled** hers away and **put both her hands over her head** as if **stretching her back**.

Fred **looked up** at the clock on the wall. He **looked to the left and then to the right**. "We'll be late for Bingo if we don't leave right now", he said. He didn't know what else to say. He knew he had almost **grabbed** her hand. He wished he just had done so. *(Who initiated the first touch of the one you married? How about your first kiss?)*

The Bingo hall was crowded as usual and they practically **ran** in. Helen, the caller, did not like anyone to be late. She usually **scowled** the entire time and **glared** at those who were. *(Do you like Bingo? Did you ever win big at Bingo? Do you like crowds?)*

Fred **pulled** out the chair for Martha and she **sat** down. She **nodded** at him and **smiled.** Then she **laughed**. It turned out to be their lucky night! Well, maybe not so much with the Bingo winnings, but they both knew now that they could be more than friends. Fred **twirled his ankles** and **tapped his heels together**! Yes, this indeed was his lucky night! BINGO!

          Charlotte Saben, ADC, AP-BC

Jake **raked** the soil in the garden. He **chopped** with his hoe. He hated the weeds that popped up! But he **loved** to garden. *(hug yourself!)* He **bent** down to **smell** the onion tops strutting proudly in a line. He **breathed in and out** several times. He loved the smell of the fresh outdoor air…and onions! *(Do you enjoy gardening? What did you grow? What did it smell like? When you think of your garden, what comes to your mind first?)*

Mattie, his wife, not so much! She was more of an indoor type. She loved to **play the piano,** and **wash the clothes**, and cook! She **stirred** the stew meat and **tossed** the veggies in the pan. She was glad Jake liked to garden. It was nice to have fresh veggies. But she still did not like the smell of onions and dirt! She **made a face** to show her distaste! *(What could cause you to make a disgusting face?) (Did you ever play an instrument? What was your favorite household chore?)*

Suddenly Jake came **running** towards the door! He was **accentuating his vowels** again and **waving his arms** wildly. What in the world made him do that?

Mattie **looked to the left and then to the right**. She **looked down…and then up**. That's when she saw the problem!

They were **flying** all around, making **buzzing** sounds. BEES! They were **chasing** Jake who was now doing a **jig** as he **raced** to the house. Mattie wasn't sure what to do. She started to **open** the door. But she didn't want the bees inside! She didn't want Jake stung either! *(Have you ever been chased by bees?)*

Suddenly she began to **laugh**. She watched as Jake **side-stepped** the door and **reached up** for the towel hanging on the clothes line. The automatic sprinklers had saved Jake a lot of pain! He **rolled his ankles** one at a time and **bent** to wipe the mud off his shoes! *(Make gestures like sprinklers with your fingers & arms.)*

He **rolled his neck** in a semi-circle and then back again! He was very thankful for those sprinklers even though he had recently ranted and cussed about them! *(Raise your fists like you are angry and make an angry face!)* *(Have you ever had trouble adjusting to some new gadget?)*

Jake **kicked** at the dirt as he **knocked** on the door. Mattie **smiled** at him through the glass. He still looked cute to her…especially all wet! She **blew him a kiss** and **pointed** at the empty basket on the picnic table. *(If you were a garden, what would grow in you?)*

Jake **nodded**, **shuddered**, **wiped** himself with the towel and **walked** over to **pick up** the basket. He **reached up** and picked the ears of corn on the stalks on the side of the garden.

They would **eat** well tonight! But he wasn't so sure about those sopping wet bees! At least they are gone...and all is well...because without those bees, Jake's garden would not get pollinated! He just needed to stay out of their way! *(A discussion of gardening or pollination might fit here! Or even planting some seeds, etc. Let them touch dirt, plants, veggies, etc.)*

Charlotte Saben, ADC, AP-BC

It was "Girls' Day Out" between Pearl, Phoebe, and Naomi. The three had been best of friends since high school and that was a long time ago! They left Carl, Troy, and Jim at one of their homes to **watch** a game or lie, or talk about their **fishing** and **hunting** expeditions. Not that some of it wasn't true…maybe. *(**Make motions like reeling and shooting, etc. and then** share some stories of sporting adventures**.**)*

The ladies **walked** briskly down the sidewalk, although "briskly" was not what it used to be. Naomi **swung** her cane around as if making it **dance** and boldly **marched** ahead. She had always liked showing off! *(Do you have any long-term friends? Share a little about them. If not, who was your best friend?)*

Pearl **pushed** her walker and **grasped** the handlebars firmly. She stopped and **opened and closed her hands several times.** Then she **moved each finger gently to the thumb one at a time**. This always seemed to loosen them up so she didn't loosen her grip. She had no desire to fall. She **made a face** recalling the last time that happened! She looked like she had been in a **boxing** match. Her husband, Troy dreamed of being a professional boxer, but he had never pursued it. *(Did you or a family member ever pursue a dream? Leave one unfulfilled? Share.)*

Phoebe stopped to **sit** on a bench. She didn't used devices to help her walk, but she tired easily. She **bent down** to examine whatever it was on the bottom of her shoe that made her feel like she had to **lift her legs really high**. She **pulled off** a gooey piece of gum with her Kleenex. Then she **pushed her torso back up, using her arms on her knees.** This **stretched** her back. She learned that somewhere. She **raised her arms in the air** and pretended to **fling** the Kleenex and offending gum onto the sidewalk. Then she **tossed** it into a nearby trash can. How easy that was! Why doesn't everybody just do that? *(What are some societal changes you dislike? How do you help keep the community clean?)*

"Yuck! I was people would be more careful!" She practically **yelled** it so perhaps the offending party would hear.

She **made circles with her ankles** as she sat. She **moved her feet up and down.** She **clicked her heels together and then her toes.** She **rolled her neck** and **looked both to her left and then her right.** No one seemed to notice her. Probably no one cared. The world just wasn't what it used to be! Her thoughts made her sigh deeply. She **breathed in and out** several times. She was glad she had good friends.

The three started down the sidewalk again, only to have to **shuffle to the side** to avoid a **bicyclist!** *(Pedaling motions like riding a bike)* They weren't supposed to ride on the sidewalk! There was even a bike lane here! Naomi **shook her fist** at the rider. Yep! This world just wasn't the same as when they were young!

Pearl **pointed** to the dress in the store window. "Look at that!" she declared. "That looks just like the prom dress I wanted about sixty some years ago! Daddy wouldn't let me, because it was too sexy he said!"

"You should get it now", Phoebe said. "Troy would really like that!"

"Oh no! I've got MUCH sexier clothes than that now! But don't you dare ask Troy! He would never admit it!" The three **laughed out loud** to the point of tears.

"And lookie over there!" This time it was Naomi who **spotted** something. "That purse!" She **held her arm out and made swinging motions.** They all tried it.

"Looks like the one you carried in high school. The one you beat up Jack Witherspoon with!" This comment brought on even more laughter. They **held their sides.** *(Share a funny memory from school days.)*

"We better go on in this store before we all fall down!" said Pearl. "LOOK! It has a soda fountain! Why, I'll be! Maybe the times haven't changed so much after all!"

"Maybe not" said Naomi. "But the prices sure have!"

"Aw! But look!" They all **glanced over their shoulders** to see a handsome young man behind the counter. They **winked** at each other. "We still got what it takes to know a good thing when we see one!" They **smiled broadly, winked** at the soda jerk and ordered big ice cream sodas! Yum! *(Make tongue on lips movements like "mmmm")* *(What is your favorite treat?)*

Charlotte Saben, ADC, AP-BC

Bill woke up, **sat up**, and **stretched his arms over his head**. He **yawned widely**. He **looked to the right and then to the left**. He **looked up and down**. He **rolled his neck around** until his eyes caught a glimpse of the clock.

"Whoa, Nellie!" He exclaimed. "I slept longer than I should have! The cow needs **milking** and the eggs need **gathering!**" *(Do you tend to over-sleep?)*

"What? Did you say something?" Nellie **rolled her eyes** as she **sat up** on the side of the bed. She **bent over** to **pull** her slippers on.

"What'd you say?" Bill asked.

"I asked what YOU said." Nellie was always a little grumpy in the morning. She **rolled her ankles in circles** and **wiggled her toes** before she settled her feet cozily in the slippers.

"It's later than I thought." Bill said. "Gotta get **moving!** Ole Bessy's calling me." He **walked** to the door and **opened** it.

"Wait, Bill!" Nellie said. "You're living in yesterday! We sold the farm and moved here to retire! We haven't got chickens and cows any more, Bill." Nellie **made a sad face** when she said this. She liked living on the farm. "All we have to do today is **drive** over to Carl and Mary's to **fish** in their new pond." *(Do you remember your first home, where you started your family?)*

"I thought they were gonna barbeque!" Bill **made several faces**. He wasn't sure he wanted Carl OR Mary to **cook. (Make motions like you are tossing a salad, stirring a pot, flipping burgers, etc.)** Last time they cooked had been an adventure he would like to forget!

"I think they know we didn't like their style." Nellie **nodded** her head and **smiled.** Bill **closed the door** and **opened and closed his hands** several times. He would like to **punch** the boxing ball, but they sold that too. He **sighed and breathed in and out** several times. He **stomped** into the kitchen. He **reached one arm out** to retrieve the frying pan. Nellie isn't a morning person. She never **cooked** breakfast. Bill missed the fresh eggs and milk. He **reached his other arm out** and pretended to balance the milk can on it. He missed the farm. He **made circles with both arms and flapped like a chicken.** No one could see him anyway. He put the frying pan back and **reached** for the cereal box. He **ate slowly** and then he **ate quickly**. Nellie **danced** into the room. She had to **move her feet quickly** or she would fall **asleep** standing up! She never was a morning person. Even on the farm! *(Are you a morning person? What time do you get up?)*

Bradley, the tom cat that adopted them **brushed** against her leg and she **swooshed him away with her hands**. He **leaped** up on Bill's lap. Bill **stroked** his fur. He **purred**.

"I think I've got an idea!" Bill declared.

"'Bout time!" Nellie retorted humorously.

"Let's **drive** over to Carl and Mary's and **wave** and then keep **driving** 'til we find farmland. Then we can **breathe it in deeply**. Maybe we can even find some fruit to **pick!"** *(What animals might they see at the farm? What would it smell like? Sound like? Feel like? Have you ever lived on a farm? Did you like it? Why/not?)*

"I hope it's lemons. I want to make lemonade." Nellie **made a lip-smacking motion with her mouth** and **blew a kiss** at Bill. "I think that's a great idea!"

"Then we can **stop** at Carl and Mary's on the way back and trade some fruit for fish! And of course, visit a while. That Mary sure can **talk, especially with her hands!"** *(Do you talk with your hands? Have you ever studied sign language?) **(This could be a good time to learn some sign language!)***

"Let's go!" Nellie **put on her sweater** and practically **skipped** to the car!

Charlotte Saben, ADC, AP-BC

Wendell **tapped** the screen gingerly. He already had **opened** up sites he hadn't meant to. His grandson, Tyler warned him about that. He **made a face**! This was NOT as easy as people say! He had just mastered his cell phone and his old computer and now this new-fangled toy had invaded his home! *(Have you ever had a device that puzzled you? What did you do?)*

Tyler said it was important for him to learn this. Wendell wasn't so sure about that. He **opened and closed his hands** several times to loosen them up. Then he **moved each finger to the thumb with a pinching motio**n. Perhaps that would make him more dexterous! He **reached** for his glasses on the shelf and **wiggled** himself in his wheelchair. According to Tyler the world was at his fingertips. *(Do you think the world is at your fingertips with a computer and the Internet? Why?)*

He **heard** the ringing of the Skype call that Tyler was trying to connect. But he didn't know how to **pull** it up.

"Hello! Hello! I can't figure this thing out!" At that point, **he accentuated his vowels** and **shook his fists**! "Don't want to miss Tyler's call but don't know why I have to use this dumb computer just because he wants to **see** me. He should come visit in person!" *(Do you appreciate calls or would you prefer personal visits?)*

Mona **nodded her head**. She agreed. Kids use technology to keep from face-to-face communication in her opinion. But one must keep up with the times! She **rolled her neck around** and **looked to the right and to the left**; and **then up and down.** She could never **sit** for hours in front of a thing like that! But it was good for Wendell to feel connected no matter how he had to do it. *(Do you think technology affects communication in a negative way? Positive Way? Why/not?)*

Wendell **kicked** at the table and **rolled his ankles** around. He **tapped his feet** to the beat of some music he had managed to evoke out of the computer. Tyler rang again. *(What is your favorite music?)*

Wendell **pushed** as many icons and keys as he could with none of them producing Tyler. "Humph!" he said. "I'm just gonna **call** him with this!" He **reached** in his pocket and **pulled out** his phone. *(Do you think people should call more than email or text? Which is better and when?)*

Just then Mona **sprinted** across the room. She **clasped her hands together** and **put her arms in the air**. To Wendell she looked like an Asian goddess doing a **dance.** *(Have you ever seen a ballet? From another country? What did you like/dislike?)*

But to Mona, it was just the start of her yoga routine. She **brought her arms to her side** and repeated this movement. She **breathed in and out** several times. She **closed her eyes** and tried to block out the world, which, at the moment only consisted of Wendell and Charlie, the dog. She **moved her arms up as she breathed in and down as she exhaled.** She **stretched her legs** and **leaned forward to stretch her back.** She **imagined** herself in her favorite place which was a private loge in the theater. She **closed her eyes** and envisioned herself **dancing** on the stage. Then, she was **singing** and **playing the piano!** How she truly wished she had pursued that dream! *(Do you have a dream you wish you had pursued? Tell us about it. Why didn't you go for it? What did you learn from it?)*

She began to **sway with her arms in the air.** Perhaps she was a palm tree **bending** toward the earth in a gentle but brisk breeze! Suddenly she **jolted** to attention! She **heard** the music! She **heard the violins** and **the tubas**, and the **drums**. And her favorite: the oboe! *(make motions like you are playing these instruments and/or put your hand to your ears for the word "heard".)* Somehow Wendell was listening to classical music! What a wonder! *(Do you and your spouse/roommate like the same music? Did you ever play an instrument?)*

She **skipped** back into the room just as he **frowned** and **clicked it off!** "Darn!" he said!

"Hello! Grandpa? I can see you!"

"Tyler? How did I manage to connect to you?"

"Perseverance!" Tyler replied.

"No. Dumb luck and **pushing** and **poking** everything around!" Mona just had to tell it the way she saw it.

Tyler and Wendell and even Mona had a good **chat t**hat day. And Tyler assured them that they would, indeed, some day master their new new-fangled toy! *(Do you think it is possible to keep learning new things? Do you like technology? How has it improved your life?)*

Charlotte Saben, ADC, AP-BC

Don **pressed** his fingers to the button. He **laughed** as he **pushed** it. He hoped he didn't look too funny. He only wanted to make Georgia **smile.** He **tapped his feet,** one at a time as he waited impatiently. Then he **knocked** on the door. And he **pounded** on the door. He **turned his head to the left and to the right**, trying to see in the window on the door. He **looked up** and then he **looked down**. He knew Georgia was in there! He could smell the liver and onions and he knew she wouldn't leave that on the stove alone! *(Do you like liver and onions? What does it smell like to you? What do you like to eat?)*

Meanwhile, Georgia **stirred** the pot. She **washed her hands** and **dried them** on a towel. Then she **shook her head** and **walked** to the door. She **peeked** through the window, **blinking** her eyes. She **shook her head** again. She figured it was Don. Silly man! But he certainly didn't look like the Don she knew. *(Have you ever dressed up in disguise to fool someone? For Halloween or a Costume party?)*

She **opened the door slowly** and carefully. It was possible that it was NOT Don. She couldn't believe she was doing this. She **kicked** at the screen which made the dog, Buster **bark.** *(Share about a dog you had. Do you like the name Buster for a dog? Would you open the door?)*

Don looked ridiculous! He **laughed out loud** and then Georgia knew it was him! *(How did she know?)* He **made face** at her, but she refused to respond.

"Come on in, Donald!" she said. "You look absolutely ridiculous! What were you thinking?"

Don didn't answer the question, but instead **stomped** through the door and into the kitchen. He **reached up** in the cupboard to get a glass. He **turned on the facet** and helped himself to a **drink**. He **stretched** his arms high in the air and **flapped** them like a chicken.

"Good thing I'm not a real chicken. You might be cooking me instead of that cow liver!" Don was usually melodramatic and today was no different. *(What is your favorite food? Do you have a special recipe? Tell me how it smells, looks, etc.)*

He **reached his arms behind his shoulders** and tried to **roll them in circles**. He **rolled his shoulders forward and backward**. He **pulled** the cloak off his shoulders and removed his disguise. He **squeezed his hands closed and opened** them again. He **stepped to the side** and **rolled his ankles in circles**. His attempts to make Georgia **laugh** went largely unnoticed. Humph!

He **sat** down at the table and began **writing rapidly** on a piece of paper. He did feel silly. But he would never let Georgia know that. He had ignored the other drivers who **honked** and **waved** at him as he **drove** by in his disguise. Now he **worried** that someone might recognize his car and discover who he is! *(Make a worried face. Make other emotional faces. Wring your hands and other worried gestures.) (Were you ever concerned about what others might think of you? How do you show worry?)*

Don **made circular motions with his feet** before he **stood up** again. He **dropped** the paper on the floor and **bent over** to **pick it up**.

RIPPP! What was that? Don **looked surprised**.

And Georgia **laughed**! She **roared**! She **bent over** in laughter and **rolled her sides**. Don had indeed made her **smile**! (What do YOU think happened?) *(Share an embarrassing moment from your life!)*

Charlotte Saben, ADC, AP-BC

Jan **walked briskly** to the pavilion. She had wanted to reserve one, but Fred had said no. He always **shook his head** and **rolled his eyes** when he disagreed with someone. Then he usually **rolled his neck around** and **turned his head from side to side.** Jan knew it was useless to argue when he was this way. *(What gestures or reactions do you or your spouse use when disagreeing?)*

Fortunately, a pavilion was available! There was only one left! She **looked up.** The sky was a pretty blue with wispy clouds **dancing** around the sunlight. She **looked down.** There were ants swarming under the table! She **stomped her feet** trying to eliminate many of them. *(Have you had to get rid of ants? How?)*

Fred sauntered up, **walking slower** than usual. He loved being outdoors, but things weren't like they used to be. He wanted to blame the "things", but he realized that it was HE who was not quite like he used to be. He **waved** at some kid **riding his bike** on the sidewalk. It wasn't exactly meant to be a friendly greeting. That kid should be in school, not **riding** on the sidewalk. Fred **shook his fist** at the kid's back. He **flexed his fingers** and **opened and closed his hands several times.** His hands were getting stiffer. In the old days he would have used more gestures! Just as well...kids don't respect their elders any more. *(Do you think society has changed with respecting elders' issues? Is this good or bad?)*

Jan **shook the tablecloth** and **spread** it out. She **patted** down the sides. Darn wind! Fred **bent down** and **picked up** a rock. He practically **tossed** it onto the table. Bang! Jan **jumped** and **made a face** at Fred. There were better ways to do things! *(How do you react when someone does something differently than you?)*

Fred **stretched** and **yawned.** He **held his hands in the air** and **swayed** like the trees in the breeze. That always helped him ignore Jan!

Jan **muttered** under her breath and then **sighed deeply.** She **breathed in and out** several times. That always helped HER ignore Fred! They both **smiled.** They'd been together so long; they just learned when to ignore each other! *(Do you think ignoring someone is good or bad? Why? How would you handle this situation?)*

Jan **tossed the salad** while Fred mimicked her, **rolling his wrists around rapidly.** He **sat** on the bench while she prepared the picnic. He **rolled his ankles** around. He hated to admit it, but they weren't what they used to be either!

He **kicked** at a piece of bread being carried by ants. At least he wasn't being stormed by pigeons! In the old days…he would have…Fred decided not to reminisce about something he couldn't completely remember. Instead, he **flapped his arms like a bird**. He knew that would get Jan's attention. These days, doing silly things for attention was about the best entertainment he had! He missed the **dancing, throwing the horseshoe, swinging** the golf club. Yes, indeed, things weren't the same as they used to be! But he could still do them all in his mind! *(What do you think about doing that you used to enjoy? Would you try it if you could?)*

And, he also had to admit that Jan was still a great cook! He **ate** with both hands but **drank** his lemonade slowly. He **puckered**. Well, maybe her lemonade making skills were being challenged…just a little! *(Name your favorite picnic food. Sense it)*

He **tapped his feet** and **rubbed** and then **patted** his tummy. These days he filled it up quicker. He **watched** a young couple **stroll** down the path.

Jan was busy **packing up** the leftovers. She **tossed** a few crumbs to the birds. Might as well! Fred was acting like one a little while ago! She **sat down** beside Fred and **reached up** to straighten his hair. She **touched** his face. He was a good man. He was strong. This time she **squeezed his muscles**, so he **flexed them** the way he had when she was young and impressionable. *(How did you feel?)*

She **hugged** him. He **tapped her on the shoulder** and **put his arm around her.** They were together forever! They were a team! They both **opened their mouths** wide and **recited their exaggerated vowels.** This was their secret code for happiness! They **blew kisses** to each other. That was as far as it goes in public! Fred **marched** to the car and **did a side-step jig**. He couldn't wait to get home. There are a few things that never change! *(What things never change for you?)*

Charlotte Saben, ADC, AP-BC

John **stuck out his toe** and **rolled his ankles**. He gingerly **put his toe in the water.** He liked this pool all right, but their version of "heated" didn't necessarily agree with his. He **shook his head**. That was to be expected since the "their" represented numerous city employees. John had once been one, so he knew how it went down. He **sat down** on the edge of the pool and **tapped his feet** in the water. He **made swooping motions with his arms**, splashing Ellen as he **circled them** in the water. (*What jobs have you had? What "secrets" did your colleagues hold?*)

"I guess it's warm enough." He thought aloud. (*Do you like cold water? Describe the perfect temperature to swim in.*) (*What is the perfect "pool"?*)

"Just what do you think you are doing, there, Mister?" Ellen **shook her finger** at him. Then she **moved her fingers separately each to the thumb**. And each **pointing**, at some point, at John! She **made faces** at him. (*Does it feel good or bad to be splashed in a pool? Have you splashed someone?*)

John **rolled his eyes** as he **jumped** in the water. "Brrr!" The first touch is always a little shocking! He ignored Ellen. She was new in town. He had heard rumors. He **hugged** himself and **rubbed his arms**. Then he **patted himself on the back**! He had taken his first dip in the winter! (*Have you swum in winter? What does the water feel like? Demonstrate your favorite swimming stroke.*)

Ellen **swam** closer to John. She had heard rumors too! In fact, John had quite a reputation! Not that it was a bad one. Ellen **kicked her feet**, splashing John. There! They were even! (*Have you heard or spread rumors? Were you ever the victim of one? How did it feel? What emotions did you express?*)

John **turned his head to right and then to the left.** Where did she go? Ellen was **making wide circles with her legs and arms** and virtually **spinning** in circles!

John **made breast-stroke motions** and **dove** under the water. He came up, **breathing deeply**. He **took several deep breaths** and **raised his arms in the air**.

Smack! Uh-Oh! John had managed to **backhand** Ellen. It was an accident! She **swam** to the ladder and **pulled herself up** and out of the pool. She had to check her nose! She had just had it "modified" this year. She **patted her face** and **opened and closed her hands several times**. That part didn't make sense to John. But then, he had never understood women! *(Do you know anyone who had "plastic surgery"? How do you feel about face lifts and such?)*

"I… I… I am so sorry, Ma'am!" John sort of **stuttered**. He **accentuated his vowels** under his breath and **prayed** she would not make a big deal out of this. *(Do you think people find too many excuses to sue others? Why or why not?)*

Ellen **ran** to the ladies' room and examined her face. There really was nothing to show. She **looked up and she looked down**. Her neck felt fine too. No whiplash even! Might as well accept his feeble apology!

Ellen **walked** back to the edge of the pool. She was intrigued by what she had heard about John. He was a decent man. AND he was single! Maybe she had a chance!

"It's all okay!" Ellen sort of **yelled** it because of the kids **splashing** in the background. They were **squealing and laughing**. She preferred age-restricted pools, but knew the kids were at least not causing trouble elsewhere.

"Whew!" John said. "Thank you! I really didn't **see** you at all!" *(Have you been involved in an accidental collision while doing a sport?)*

"Well, how about we say you owe me a coffee and call it good?"

John **nodded his head**. That was better than getting sued!

"And I suppose you would like that immediately?" John was hoping to get this whole thing over. He **scratched his head**. He remembered the rumors. But then, he remembered who had told him the rumors too! Rumors be gone! Might as well give her a chance to be a friend. *(Have you discovered a new friend by ignoring rumors?)*

Ellen and John **chatted** as they **drank their coffee** and found they had a lot in common. Yes, indeed! They would be good friends after all.

Charlotte Saben, ADC, AP-BC

Lucy was a very superstitious person. She lived life very carefully. She started her **walk** every day with **stretching.** And today the neighborhood black cat had **crossed** her path! Yes, it **ran** right in front of her! She **jumped** straight up in her chair where she had just **bent down** to tie her shoe. Now there would be bad luck unless she found an antidote. Her husband, Carl, told her to ignore the cat and just **kick** the **door shut** so as not to see such things! Perhaps since it was outside, and she was inside, the omen would be nullified. *(Are you superstitious? What about? Share experiences where things happened to convince you.)*

She **got up** from the chair by **pushing her hands on her knees** and rising. This seemed to **stretch** her back. She **put her hands together and stretched them over her head.** She **swayed** back and forth. She **opened and closed her hands** around the rabbit's foot that was in her pocket. She wouldn't go on a **stroll** without that thing! Carl thought that was silly and **made a face**. *(Do you have a lucky charm? Do you believe in them?)*

Lucy didn't care! Carl seemed to forget **slipping** when he **walked** under that ladder. He was in a hurry as usual, and tried to **side-step** through the ladder rather than **climb** around. That is NOT a good thing to do. The paint pan **dropped** and Carl had found himself covered in paint! His **legs sprawled** out as he went **down.** How he could forget that is a wonder! Lucy **shook her head** and then **rolled her eyes and then her neck.** She **looked to the right and then to the left.** One can never be too cautious! *(Tell me about some cautious things we ought to do. Have you ever had paint spilled on you? What did it feel, smell, like?)*

As she looked up, she **spotted** the tiniest of dark clouds. "Oh no!" she thought. "It looks like rain!" *(Do you know someone who sees the darkest things first?)*

"Looks fine to me! Lots of fluffy clouds!" Carl retorted. Lucy hadn't realized her thoughts had escaped her mouth. She **put her hand over her mouth**, but it was already too late! Carl had **pulled** out the umbrella to tease her. He **smiled broadly** as he **opened** it. *(Is it bad luck to open an umbrella indoors? Why or why not?)*

"No! Don't do that in here!" Lucy **screamed**. "Everyone knows not to **open** an umbrella indoors!" This was definitely NOT her lucky day!

She **ran** outside as fast as she could! And without any warning, she **stepped** on, and then **tripped** on a crack in the sidewalk! But she didn't fall! Must be that rabbit's foot! Or maybe the St. Christopher medal she had worn ever since the 70's. *(Do you remember any crazes from your youth? Your children's youth? Tell me what you remember about the 70's)*

She **waved** to Carl who was standing in the window. She **gave him a "thumbs up!"** He looked kind of silly **standing** inside with that umbrella! She **laughed** out loud!

Lucy knew she was somewhat of a pessimist. She couldn't help it. She seemed always see things half-empty. She was drawn to the dark side. She **sighed.** She **heaved her shoulders and then rolled them forward and backward.** She wished she could change, but at seventy-five, it wasn't likely! She **took several deep breaths,** trying to feel the positive energy in the air. *(What is a pessimist? Are you one? Are you an optimist? Share experiences that molded your choices.) (Let's take a moment and* **breath in and out** *and* **take in some positive energy***.)*

She **moved her arms in small and then big circles** and imagined herself **flying** like a bird. She could be free! But, alas! Lucy was Lucy and knew she couldn't **fly.** *(If you could fly, what would you be? What color? How big? Name some things that fly both living and mechanical.)*

She **stomped** back into the house. Forget the longer **walk** today! She **sat down at the piano and began to play**. The music calmed her down. **Humming** along helped too. Carl gave her a **hug** and **smiled**. She didn't need to change! He was an incurable optimist and she a pessimist…a perfect match! And sometimes Carl admitted that her premonitions came true. So he heeded her advice frequently. That's why he loved her so! *(Were/Are you and your spouse/significant other opposites? How? Do you find that good or bad? If not opposites, is that good or bad? Why? Do you play an instrument? What music calms you? What else calms you? Remember we are all unique and special…**HUG YOURSELF!**)*

Charlotte Saben, ADC, AP-BC

Alice, Jenny, and Susan enjoyed shopping. Their weekly trip to the mall was about to begin. Alice **stretched her arms in the air** and **breathed deeply**. She loved shopping but was determined to get into those size 8s! She put her **arms over her head and brought her hands together.** Then she **stretched her arms to the side and made circles…starting small and getting bigger**. She really hated exercises but wasn't about to let Susan wear a smaller size than she did. So, she **bent down to touch her toes**. Up and down…several times. She **ran in place** for about three seconds. There! That ought to do it! She **walked** to the pantry, **opened it** and **pulled** out a box of donuts! She rewarded herself for exercising. (*Do you reward yourself for doing something? Do you defeat your plan by your rewards? Share about this) (Do you compare yourself to others? In what ways?*)

Jenny could care less about what size she wore! Susan and Alice had always been smaller than she was! She **shook her feet** while she sat on the edge of her bed. She **rolled her ankles** and **touched her heels and then her toes**. She was the shoe expert! No matter what size she wore, Jenny had the most fashionable shoes available. She **tapped her toes** on the carpet. Today she would find a new pair! A new color! A new style! Her feet had long ago gotten used to new shoes. She hardly noticed the pain any more. She **kicked** at her husband's shoe blocking the door to the closet. Silly man! Buys the same pair of shoes in only two colors and one at a time! Ridiculous! But she loved him anyway. She **blew a kiss** into the air. She was sort of glad he was on a **fishing** trip with his brother…and sort of not. (*How were you and your partner different? Describe your favorite shoe. How would you design a shoe?*)

Susan was gloating as she **primped** in the mirror. She **raised** one leg and **then the other.** She admired herself as she **rubbed her legs**. Then she **rolled her neck** around and **looked up and then down**. She **looked to the left and then to the right.** Darn! She looked good at any angle! **Standing** in front of that three-way mirror John had bought at the auction made her **smile broadly**.

She **made a face**, though, at the recollection of the hassle she had given him for going to auctions in the first place! Oh, well. He had forgiven her. She **opened and closed her hands several times**. She hated to admit it, but she didn't feel as strong as she used to. She **pressed each finger up against the thumbs**. They didn't move as easily as they used to! She **rubbed each nail with her thumb**s. Her friends thought she was vain. She knew she was just **fighting** that aging feeling. And John knew it too even though he called her "hot" on a regular basis. She had many moments of feeling hot, though giving it a different meaning as she **fanned herself**. She'd like to **raise** the air-conditioning but **shook her head**. That last bill was astronomical, according to John. He was a good provider so she just gave in and **fanned herself** some more.

 Her goal for the day was to get into those size 8 skinny jeans she saw at the mall. Never mind that they were purple…all the better, in her opinion. *(What is the craziest thing you or your spouse ever bought? Have you been to an auction? What did it sound, smell, feel like? Do you like to buy used items? Why or why not?) (Have you ever had to deal with aging symptoms? Can they be funny?)*

The three "girls" **walked** into the mall together and then parted. Jenny headed for the shoe store as **quickly as she could go**. Alice saw a jewelry display that had her name written all over it! She immediately **began trying on earrings**. Susan knew exactly where those purple skinny jeans were, so she practically **skipped** into that store. *(What dept. would you head to?)*

They had their own measure of vanity, for sure, but that was part of being female…well, maybe of just being human! She **laughed out loud** at the thought while imaging her husband **showing off his muscles**. *(Where do you think you or your family might be vain?)*

The time **flew** by and the girls had hardly time to **relax** and **drink** some tea. Sodas were no-no's! They all **took some deep breaths**, in and out, and tried to not stress at the thought of the traffic. *(What stresses you? Does deep-breathing help? What does?)*

"You know, "Alice said. "They used to tell us at yoga class to **imagine a favorite place while deep breathing…**Well, this is mine! The mall!" She **looked around** and **spanned her hands** as if presenting it in front of an audience.

"Well," said Susan. "Mine is home with the grandchildren."

"I'm really torn," **cried** Jenny. "I **love** my home and family, but wow! This is my favorite home away from home! Well, except maybe the beach…or Disneyland! *(Where is your favorite place away from home?) (Why is it your favorite? What appeal does it hold for you?)*

The sound of an announcement brought them all **running** out the door. There was no emergency, just a reminder of the time **flying** by. *(Have you ever stayed too long shopping? Hunting, fishing, etc.?)*

"See ya next week!" Susan **yelled** as she **bent down** to check the license plate on a car. *(Do you or did you have trouble finding your car in a parking lot?)*

Charlotte Saben, ADC, AP-BC

"Yep!" said Alice. "Be here or be…near?" They all **laughed**.

"You got it!" replied Jenny. "I'll be here with bells on my new shoes!" She did a **little jig** as she **climbed** into her car. They all **waved** good bye. They cherished their friendship and memories. *(Tell me about your best memories of friendship. Who is your current best friend? How do you make friends?)*

Seth wasn't entirely sure he wanted to do this. Anna was so excited that she was **dancing** around the room **kicking** furniture along the way. She **raised her arms** in the air and **twirled** them like a ballerina. Seth **looked to the right and to the left**. Even inside the house he was afraid someone might be **watching**. *(Make motions like you are looking such as hands to eyebrows)*. It wasn't that Anna couldn't **dance**, it's just that HE couldn't and she wants him to practice with her! *(Can you dance? Did you used to like it? With whom? Favorite dance style?)*

Seth **pouted** and **made several faces**, ending his antics with a **smile**. He **loved** Anna and fifty years ago he would have **jumped** at this opportunity to escort her to the prom! He **stretched out his arms** and **flapped them like a bird**. He **squawked** like one too. This usually made Anna **laugh**. But today she ignored him. She **rolled her eyes** and then her **neck**. She **walked** to the bedroom with a **smile** on her face. *(Have you gone to some event just because someone wanted you to? What was it? How did you feel about it?)*

He tried to imagine them as teenagers. He **shook his head** sadly, remembering that they had not been able to attend their last high school dance. He had gotten called into the war by an enlisting date error. And off he **marched** to the Army. He remembered that she had **made** a red beaded dress. *(Move fingers like doing beadwork)*. He **opened and closed his hands several times** realizing how dexterous her hands must have been back then. He knew now that he could and would do this for her! *(Did you make your own clothes? Did you do needlework or beadwork? What was hard? Easy? How did it make you feel when it was done?)*

They had received the invitation two months ago. Some old high school buddies were hosting a Senior Prom. It was ironic that they had managed to never leave their home town! Well, not forever anyway. Nor had Seth and Anna. *(What is your home town? How long did you live there? Why did you move away?)*

Anna and Seth had lived many places. The military even sent them across the sea! They had loved **surfing** and **swimming** along the coastlines! Anna was fearless! She even liked to **dive** off cliffs in the day! *(Share an adventure you had...or one you wish you had tried.)*

They had many adventures. They had **hunted** for deer and elk together. They had **bicycled** over mountains! They **milked** cows. Anna never complained one bit! And the final adventure was the road back to where it all began! The road back home! *(Have you milked a cow? Hunted for deer? Biked a long way?)*

And now, the evening has come for the big event. It is Seth's opportunity to take Anna to the prom! He **stomped** into the bathroom and began to **shave**. He **took a shower** and put on the suit she had bought at the church rummage sale. Lucky for her, it fits! Anna said she found herself the perfect dress to compliment him! He thought she complimented him no matter what she wore. *(Describe the perfect dress!)*

Anna sat on the bed and **clicked her toes and heels together**. She wanted to make sure her ruby slippers would not fall off. What a rummage sale that had been! She **combed her hair**, **smeared on her lipstick** (Seth's favorite color) and **posed** in the mirror. Somehow she didn't mind all the wrinkles it revealed because she knew each one was preceded by a **smile**! *(Do you focus on the smiles of your life?)*

Seth **put his hands on his cheeks** and **gasped** aloud! Was it really? Could it be?

Anna appeared in a gorgeous red beaded dress…just like the one she had made so many years ago! She **winked** at him and **tossed her head** proudly! It was quite an accomplishment to be able to **squeeze** into it at her age! He **put his hand on his hip**, **stuck out his elbow** for her to take. What a proud man he was! And what a lovely prom surprise! *(Do you think it was the same one she made?)*

They **walked** out the door ready to do the **two-step**, or any of those other **fancy steps** they cannot recall the names of anymore. But they never forgot the **moves!**

(Share about a dance, date, or fun thing you did with spouse or family)

Karl **collected** all the money and **put it in an envelope in his pocket**. Everybody but Steven bet that they would **catch** the biggest fish today. Steven never bet on anything. No one asked why. They just accepted him. The **wind was blowing** and the **waves were choppy**, but Karl and his fearless men were determined to keep their charter boat commitment. The clouds were **rolling** across the early morning sky threatening **rain**. No matter. They were going out anyway. *(Would you have gone? Have you ever gone deep sea fishing?) (Why did Steven not participate?)*

The captain expressed little concern. His main thought was that the fish might not be **biting** and he wanted no complaints at the end of the day. All on board **agreed**. But Ralph had to **scowl** just a little. All the men started **making crazy faces**. It was a guys' out day, after all! Karl **opened and closed his hands** several times. This weather made them a little stiffer than he liked. He **moved each finger to the palm of his hand and then to his thumb**. That ought to loosen things up a bit. Karl was the one who charted the boat and he wasn't about to be deterred by stiff hands. He checked his pole, reel, and line. Everything seemed perfect. His stomach felt the effect of the waves immediately. He **grabbed it and took a deep breath.** *(Do you get seasick? Carsick? Airsick? What do you do?)*

Soon the captain cut the engine and announced his sonar had found a school of rock cod. The boat **rocked** suddenly and Karl had to **side step** to keep from falling. He **walked** to the other side **gingerly**, trying to keep from **sliding**. Karl **dropped** his line over the side of the boat. He wondered why the other men were **huddled** across the boat where he had just been. Oh, well. He was going to catch the biggest fish and take home the fish and the pot of money! He **tapped his pocket** to make sure it was still there. *(Share about a scary experience you had.)*

Suddenly the men dispersed and seemingly **throwing** their poles in every direction. They seemed to be confused and bothered by each other. It wasn't but a few minutes until one of them shouted loudly, "I've got it! I've got the winning fish!"

"You mean you got the FIRST fish!" Karl corrected him.

"No! This is big doozy of a fish for sure! I need help **reeling** him in!"

No one exactly **jumped t**o assist him. Partly because it was Pete. He was always overly dramatic. Partly because some had figured out the situation and had begun to **laugh** and **moan** at the same time.

Charlotte Saben, ADC, AP-BC

Meanwhile Pete was **yanking** and **jerking** the pole, **swinging his arms wildly** while trying to hold on to it. The pole bent as if the fish was **swimming** back under the boat. Pete **sidled sideways, moving his feet together** across the bottom of the boat. He was **making circles with his feet**, trying to keep up with the movement of whatever great monster was on his line.

He was **pushing** and **elbowing** people to move so his pole didn't **fly** out of his hands. *(Would you be rude in order not lose out on a big prize?)*

Suddenly five other men simultaneously let out a big **groan.** They began to **accentuate their vowels** rather than let loose with the words they wanted to say. One of them **stomped his feet** and another **kicked** the side of the boat. Two others started **sparring** with each other. The fifth sat down and **pouted**! Several more men began to **laugh.** But as they began to **reel in** their lines, they went back and forth between the laughter and the cursing.

Karl came **running** up the deck and produced a large knife. He **raised it in the air** for attention. The men began to **pull together** to **lift** their lines out of the water.

What a tangled mess! With the wind **blowing** so hard, the lines had all **drifted** together under the boat, no matter where they were **dropped**. But as the lines appeared from the water, behold! A large fish was entangled in ALL of them. The fish **struggled** for a short time and then **heaved** his last. Indeed, this would be the largest fish caught today...and it appeared ALL the fishermen were the winners! Karl would just have to give back everyone's money! What a time of selfies and other pictures and the spinning of tall tales!

There were a few small fish caught that day...with a net. But for the most part, the deep-sea fishing trip had gone with the wind! Karl didn't admit it, but when he **did the little jig**, it was because he hadn't really wanted to fish today... deep down he only wanted to be with his buddies and away from Mary's "Honey-Do" list! And chartering a deep-sea fishing boat was the only reasonable excuse she would accept. *(Name some things a Honey-do list might have on it.)*

"Rainy days and Mondays always get me down!" Ralph said it matter-of-factly with a twinkle in his eye and a lilt in his voice. "That's what the Carpenters said! And I agree! Look at that rain come down!" He **accentuated his vowels** as he **gestured** with his arms. "Birds can't even fly in this!" He **made motions like a bird with his arms**. He **made faces.**

"Time for exercise!" That was Tina! She always wants to **kick** up something or **stretch her back and arms!**

"I'd rather watch the rain" said Sheila. She **mimicked the raindrops falling** from the sky. "It's rather amusing" she said as she **swayed her arms back and forth.**

"You're too easily amused!" said Ralph. "Rain is boring. It is repetitious and gloomy! That's why it gets me down. Especially on Mondays!"

"Today is Tuesday, Ralph!" Sheila retorted as she **pretended to swing** at him. He **ducked** and **rolled his head around several times**. Rain got him down partly because of his arthritis! **He looked to the left and to the right.** Then he **looked up and down**. He wasn't particularly looking for something; he just wanted to **stretch his neck** without being obvious about it. Too late!

"Hey Ralph! Those were some good **moves,** there, Buddy!" Tina again. She was the resident activity assistant and always **begging** people to get active! What a nuisance she was to Ralph. He **stretched his arms out to his side** and **made circles in the air**. Maybe that would satisfy her and she would leave him alone.

"Way to go, Ralph!" she said. "Let's all get moving!"

"And groovin' too? Byron always had to add something!

"Sure! If you can groove, you go right ahead!" Tina replied. *(What did it mean to get "groovin' and movin'"?)*

"I think I forgot how to do THAT a LONG time ago!" Ralph said gloomily.

"I think you were never IN the groove in the first place!" Sheila needed to have the last word. She **walked briskly** towards the area Tina had set up for **exercise.** She would "get in on" anytime! She just liked to be challenged. And she liked to be reluctant. *(Describe* *how one was "in the groove".) (Do you readily join I groups or hang back? Do you like competition and/or challenge?)*

Byron smiled **broadly.** He liked Sheila. She usually says she won't participate in Tina's activity groups, initially, but then she almost always joins in. Likes to play hard-to get, he assumed.

Soon Tina had them **kicking, touching their heels together and then their toes**, and **rotating their ankles** like they were teenagers again! Well, almost. She even had the audacity to ask them to **bend** over and **touch their toes** with their hands! She did that just to show off! Or maybe she liked to hear the creaking of their backs! Byron wasn't sure. *(Does exercising make you feel younger? Why/why not?)*

"Rainy days and Mondays ALWAYS get me down!" Ralph said it again. This time he punctuated it with a **shaking of his fist**! "AND…" he **pointed** to Sheila… "I don't care if it IS Tuesday! It's still a rainy day!"

"But it rained yesterday and you didn't say a word! Why was that, Ralph?" She **glared** at him and then **laughed out loud**! "I know! It was because you got your days mixed up! You thought it was Sunday all day! No wonder you were acting so good!"

Ralph **pouted** his best pout! She was right. He got things, even days, way more mixed up than he used to. If that Church would just stop having Mass every day maybe he could get it right! He **walked,** no he **danced** across the floor to the door. At least he could still **move** better than Sheila.

"Wanna **race?**" He **winked** at her which made Byron **frown.** He **ran** a little faster, **stepping high** as he did.

"Now don't you go falling for me!" Tina **giggled** like a Junior High School girl. The **glare** Sheila gave Ralph could've **knocked** over a statue! They both **laughed** and gave themselves **hugs**. A rainy Tuesday could turn out to be fun after all! Especially if they all played…? *(What should they all play together? Or should they? What is your favorite table games? Electronic game? Physical game? Game to watch? What would YOU do on a rainy day?*

Sandy **wheeled** her chair rapidly down the hall. She was practicing for the Olympic Races they were having this afternoon. She **flung her arms out to the side and made circles** with them. She deemed herself the champion hula hoop arm wrestler in the entire community! She would show them all! She will win both the race AND the hoops for sure!

"You came down that hall way too fast!" Bobbi, THE nurse scolded. "I've told you before to slow down! You're gonna **run** into something someday. And stop **flapping your arms** about too! You could **hit** someone!" *(Do you think she was being careless or just exuberant?)*

Well, they should all keep their distance! I am the Champ!" Sandy retorted.

"You don't look nothin' like Ali!" Danny said. He liked Muhammad Ali and had posters of him on his wall. Danny **made faces** at Sandy. But she didn't see him. That was good because Danny was quite shy, especially around women. He **"put up his dukes", flexing his muscles**, and announced, "There's only one Champ!" And **taking a deep breath** so he couldn't totally be heard, he added "and it's NOT you!" *(Did you admire Ali? Why or why not?) (Do you like boxing?) (Who is a sports figure that you admire?)*

"Well, we'll just see about that this afternoon, now won't we?" Sandy **spun** her chair around as if on one wheel and **laughed**. She was quite the character. Oh, yes! If they only knew! Sandy had once been a contender for a spot in the real Olympics in Women's track and field. She mostly was a **sprinter** but had won **long jump** contests as well. She **stretched her back** and **legs** out in remembrance. She **rolled her neck both directions** and **stretched it back** as far as she could. She tried to **bend down** but only managed to **lower her chin to her chest**. How she wished she could do all those **warm-up moves** of yesteryear! Oh, yes! She really was something back then! Everyone knew her name in the entire state where she lived. Good thing she had changed it…several times…with marriages. She did not desire to relive the past in the presence of others. They wouldn't understand. *(Do you like to share about your past freely or cautiously? Why?)*

All it took was one wrong decision. She **frowned** and **shook her head** to keep the tears from forming. Even after all these years, it still stung! She **stretched her arms over her head** and **opened and closed her hands** several times. One stupid decision! It had cost her all her hopes and dreams. She **kicked** at the wall as she **rolled** down the hall…much slower.

Charlotte Saben, ADC, AP-BC

Bobbi was nice but was sort of a no-nonsense nurse. *(What do you think this terrible decision was? Have you or someone you know made any big mistakes?)*

She took several **deep breaths** and let the memories…of the good times **dance** through her head. She saw herself **running**. She was ahead! She was behind! She **pushed** herself more and was ahead again! She was **running faster** and faster, feeling free and confident! She wished she could feel that way now. She **closed her eyes tightly** and **then lightly** to recall the feel of **flying** through the air! The **run** was the key, next to the **lunge** into the air! The feel of the sand through her shoes was exhilarating! She **made leaping motions** with her legs until the nurse warned her not to **fall** out of the chair. Oh yeah! That one dumb decision… *(Have you played a sport? Ran? Jumped? How did you feel?) (If you could undo just one thing in your life, what would it be?)*

But her life had not been all bad since the day she learned she would never be in the Olympics again…not even as the alternate she had almost been once.

She **smiled** as she remembered **walking** down the aisle for the first time. Tom looked so handsome! She **blew him a kiss** from the back of the room and then a **big hug** when she said "I do!" Those days went by too fast. They **rode their bikes** together, even with two toddlers in tow. And then… *(Describe your wedding day.) OR (What do you think happened to Tom?)*

She **rolled her ankles** and **put her heels and toes together** the way she had when she had met Jake. He noticed her **fidgeting** and helped her **untangle** her fishing line! How embarrassing! He taught her how to **cast** and how to **reel** them in…just like he did to her! And then there were two more toddlers…and no more Jake!

(Do you think one marriage was happier than the other? Which? What is a clue in this story?)

She **opened the door** and **rolled** out to the garden where she could **accentuate her vowels** without disturbing anyone. **Counting to ten**, even with her fingers never calmed her down. Especially when she remembered her Bill, her hero. She started to reminisce about all the fun they had **riding** horses, but Bobbi **called** her inside for lunch. Just as well! *(Do you have a hero? Who? How did they earn the title?)*

The one stupid mistake she had made! She held regret for her whole life. It did though, kind of help to make her the sassy, fun, colorful person she was today and she did kind of like herself now. She **clicked her heels together** and said "There's no place like home…and home is where your heart is…and where you find your body at the moment!" She was looking forward to this afternoon. She was ready! *(Do you like who you are today? Give yourself a big hug and tell me why you deserve one! If you have any regrets let's squeeze them to death and then release them with a deep breath and release of hand. Now give herself an even bigger hug!)*

Joel **opened** the door to Sportsman's School. It was actually just a detached garage he had made into a training center. He **gently kicked** at Oliver, the stray dog who had made this porch his home. He **stepped over** the dog. He gave him another **nudge** as the young men would soon be here and he didn't want anyone **tripping** over Oliver. *(no actual tripping her please. Just move your feet and perhaps bend forward slightly as if catching yourself from a fall.)*

Joel's wife and mom did not like his hobby. They **frowned** and **scowled** and even **begged** him to quit. But it provided the extra income the family needed. And it served a very important purpose. No one should be hunting without the lessons on safety and laws that Joel's school provided. He taught boys (and men) how to hunt safely and purposefully. *(Do you like to hunt? Fish? What are the laws in the state you are from?)*

He would show them rifles, crossbows, fishing rods, and weapons of hunters gone before. *(Can you name some ancient weapons? Modern ones? Compare.)*

Soon the place was filling up with the young men. They **made all kinds of faces** as many **stomped** on the welcome mat while **walking** around Oliver who stayed secure at his spot. They **wandered** through the room gently **touching** the weapons.

Joel always began with a history lesson. He **pulled** a spear from its perch on the wall. He demonstrated how many hunters **hurled it through the air** to capture prey for food and clothing. He showed them clubs and knives made from stones. The prehistoric people had to be swift and quiet and very sneaky in capturing their prey with those tools. *(make actions of sneaking up on prey)*

Joel shared how our Native Americans used bows and arrows made from flint and other stones to subdue prey. They used every piece possible of the animal and valued that life in a special way. He **pulled back on the bow** and sent a plastic arrow **sailing** through the air. He **moved his fingers, one at a time, to his thumb** and back again to loosen them for the "twang".

Joel wanted the men to know, not just how to hunt, by why they want to hunt in the first place. He wanted them to be safe, and to value all life. Obviously, Joel did not have qualms about hunting, but he did have feelings about limits and boundaries. He **raised his hands above his head** and began to **sway like a tree.** The class of guys copied him. Then he stretched out his arms and **flapped like a bird.** *(What kind of bird would you be if you had to be a bird and could choose?)*

 "Feel the freedom of flight," he said. Then he had them **bend towards the floor with their arms above their heads.** *(What might it feel like? Ever been hang-gliding or parachuting? **Show video of these sports if able.**)*

"Feel the power," he said. "You are the Earth and everything in it. We all work together to sustain life." Joel **smiled** at himself. He was getting too philosophical. But he wanted to emphasize that hunting for sport should have its limits and should still respect the life of all creatures. He had them **act like bears and eagles; like fish swimming in the pond, and like deer leaping in the meadows.** *(What animal would you like to be if you had to be one? What would it feel like?)*

He **raised** a rifle to his shoulder and explained how they **kick** back at you. He **pulled the trigger** and sent a loud **BANG** ringing through the air. Everyone **plugged the ears** momentarily. **They looked left and right** at his command.

He let them **stab** foam creatures with knives, and **reel in** resistive plastic fish heavy enough to raise a sweat. He also showed videos of animals **playing** the fields and fish **swimming** in the ponds. *(What does it smell like? Feel? Sound?)*

"Now ask yourself…Why do I want to hunt?" *(Why do you think some want to hunt? Is it inbred ancestral cravings?)* "And how will I manage the carcass? How will I use the meat?" Joel always felt that if one isn't willing to either **eat** the meat or share it with someone hungry, that they should not be hunting and he made that clear. *(Do you agree with Joel? Why or why not? What other reasons might there be to go hunting? Did you ever go hunting? What did you hunt? How do you feel about hunting as a sport? How about as survival? Is it about power?)*

Charlotte Saben, ADC, AP-BC

I can't **sing**! I just can't!" Marvin didn't like attention unless it was one-on-one. He didn't like the spotlight. He **made faces** at Tessa, the Activity Director who was simply **asking** him to be in a Christmas **caroling** group. It was a "choir" in his mind and he wanted nothing to do with it! *(Do you like caroling? Being part of a group? Do you like to sing?)*

He **walked** away from her as quickly as he could. Millie **wheeled** up in her chair ready to challenge him. "Betcha can sing better than me!"

Tessa **put her hands to her ears** and **laughed.** Millie REALLY couldn't sing! But she liked to lead the group on the side, **waving her arms like a true maestro**! And, it turns out, she CAN **play the piano**! And, she likes to recruit people! She **smiles** a lot and likes to **shake hands** or **pat the backs** of everyone! Most of the time it was taken as friendliness. Millie **opened and closed her hands** several times. She hated to admit that sometimes her arthritis got to her. She would conquer! *(Did you ever play an instrument? Would you try to now? OR How do you manage challenges in life? How do you conquer?)*

"Why're you so afraid of singin' Marv?" she inquired, although she already knew the answer! He had **told** the story more times than she could **count**! But it was funny and she liked hearing it over and over. *(Do you like to hear things or movies more than once? Do you watch re-runs?)*

Marvin **kicked** at the floor and **punched his fists into the air**. "I think I already told you once…or maybe it was Myrtle…no, Betty! Anyway…I guess I can tell it one more time." He **winked** at Millie and **moved his arms in circles**.

"I was in a choir once, you see…and I was putting on my choir robe like this…" he emphasized his motions **rolling his arms in a forward motion**.

"Oh No! You ain't tellin' THAT story again, are you? Well, I guess you ARE!" Max was usually **grumpy (make grumpy faces or sounds)** so Marvin just ignored him. He **stuck his nose in the air** and started to go on…He **rolled his neck around several times** and **looked to the right and to the left**. Then he **looked up and down.** *(What do you do when friends or neighbors do things that annoy you?)*

"What's you stallin' for?" Millie could be impatient!

"Just checking to make sure there's no more grumps around!" He **stretched his arms over his head** and **swayed like a tree**. *(If you were a tree, what kind would you be? What is your favorite fruit tree? Shade tree?)*

"Cuz he can't remember his own old boring story!" Max **pouted** as he said this. He **put his hands on his hips** and **stomped his feet**, one at time of course!

"Can too!" Marvin said. "It was for a Christmas Cantata at that church Ginny also made me go to! I decided I might as well be somebody…so I joined their choir! I was **putting on that robe** like I showed you." He **made the same motions again**. "And out of nowhere, little Jimmy, the Pastor's kid, came **running** and **knocked** me clean off the stage! And I **swallowed** the gum drop in my mouth so hard I couldn't **talk**, much less **sing**." *(Have you ever been involved in an embarrassing situation? Tell us about it.) OR (Do you think children should be better monitored?)*

Millie **laughed** like she'd never heard the story before.

"And the worst part was they were **filming! (Make motions like rolling a camera, etc.)** And they wouldn't delete that part! They showed it at the All-church Christmas party! And EVERYBODY **laughed** at me! And I've NEVER been able to **sing** again! Plain and simple!" *(Do you think it was right of the choir director to play the scene at the party? Why or why not? How would you have reacted…as the victim? As a church member? OR tell us about Holiday parties you have attended. What did you like? Dislike? Any stories to share?)*

Tessa **hugged** Marvin and got out the **rhythm instruments to play** instead. ***(pretend you are using maracas, triangles, kazoos, etc. unless you have them, then get them out!)***

"Maybe we can do a kitchen band instead." Who said that? *(What is a kitchen band? Have you ever played in one? Seen one play?)*

Charlotte Saben, ADC, AP-BC

Jan **shook her head.** She knew she should have just said no, but that had always been a challenge for her. *(Is saying no to people hard for you to do? Certain people or in general? Why do you think it is or is not?)* She **looked up** at the ceiling. She **looked down** at the carpet. She did this several times trying to figure out what it was she was seeing. Was that spot on the ceiling jelly? If so, how in the world did it get there?

She **looked to the right and then to the left.** The kids were nowhere in sight. She wasn't sure if that was good or not. The spot on the carpet almost looked like blood. She **frowned.** She **made several faces**. *(Share an experience where you found something unidentifiable in your house.)*

Jan **got up** and **walked** to the sliding glass door and **pulled** it open. There they were! Oh, yeah! There they were…with the hose spraying all over, **winding like a snake** attacking the kids and the windows and the dog and his house and…oh my! Just a few minutes of **quiet breathing** had led to this disaster. *(Did you ever play in the hose or sprinkler? What other outdoor games did you play? Your children?)*

The children did not consider it disastrous at all! They were **running** and **clapping** and **jumping** up and down. They **smiled** and **laughed** out loud. They **grabbed** the hose and **sprayed it up and down**, showering Jan in the process. *(Shiver)*

She **bent down** to **pick up** the cat that was hiding, **shivering** in the corner of the patio. She missed the cat and **stood** up **rolling her shoulders.** She was angry. *(**Make an angry face or motion**).* And she was amused. *(Have you been angry and amused at the same time? What caused it? If not, do you think it is possible?)* She **stepped over** a puddle and **yanked** the hose from the children. They **bent over laughing**. She **kicked** off her soggy shoes. She **turned** the handle on the valve to shut off the water. *(Would you have punished the children? How and why?)*

Jan knew it was sort of her fault. She sent them outside on this warm day without checking for temptations that may lie around. She **sighed deeply**. The children had been a challenge all day. They had **climbed** up on the counter and spilled cereal all over the floor. Then Toby had **knocked** Jan's cup of coffee on the floor while trying to **sweep** up his mess. Then both Toby and Caroline had a **punching** match that sent Caroline **crying** and **running** to her room, **slamming** the door. *(Have you experienced times like these with children in your life?)*

It was almost time for lunch when Toby **announced** his big building accomplishment. *(Cup your hands around your mouth like you are yelling or make motions to get someone's attention.)* Indeed! He had managed to **build** a tower of over a hundred Legos! Caroline **pushed** them over which resulted in Toby **swinging** at her. She claimed it was an accident. *(Did your children have such "accidents"? How did you teach them to accept responsibility for their choices and actions?)*

So, she sent them outside to wear themselves out. She had sat quietly **breathing in and out rhythmically** and **imagining herself miles away**. That was when she came to her senses! *(Where does your mind take you?)*

She was glad she had brought that extra pair of pants she thought, as she **placed her legs into them one at a time.** Kids! No wonder her niece needed a day off!

But there had been good moments today too. Like playing Candyland and even Twister. She **crossed her legs** and **then her arms, flinging them** in the air. Twister might not be her game of choice, but it sure did make those kids **giggle.** She **opened and closed her hands several times** before **picking up** the bread. *(What games did your family play?)*

Jan **placed the sandwiches on the table** and **sat down** with the now gloomy children. Mom and Dad would think they were naughty when they saw the messy patio. Jan hadn't even noticed that the dog had **dug** mud holes in the yard as well.

Oh, well. A good lunch and story time would make the day better. *(Pretend to eat and/or read...or act out a story.)* She **drank** her now cold coffee and **smiled**. She **loved** these kids! She **rolled her ankles around** under the table and gave them each a **hug.** She was sure they would take **naps.** Surprisingly, they agreed and **skipped** off to their beds. Suspicious!

Yes, Dad would have to **clean up** the yard. But Jan would not blame the children. She would find some logical reason for the mess. She knew she could. She also knew she should have said no to babysitting. But she also knew she never would.

(What ideas might she have for explaining the mess? Did you pick up some clues in the story?)

Charlotte Saben, ADC, AP-BC

Joe **walked** to the door and **slammed** it shut. He **pulled** down the window shade hoping to block out the festivities! Joe did want to let the year pass. It had been a great year and he didn't want to take chances on a new one. It had definitely been a while since Joe had had this great of a year!

"Bah! Humbug!" He said. He **made a face**. He **made several faces** and **shook his fist** at the window. He wanted to **dance** and rejoice, but he couldn't.

Joe didn't like change at all. He knew this New Year would bring some. He would be **packing** up his things and **moving** to a care center. He **scowled** at the thought. It wasn't that he was afraid of the center. He had several friends already there. It was the thought of not being able to do what he wanted. He **opened and closed his hands several times**. They were much stiffer than last year.

He tried to **march** in place, but his knees complained loudly. He **kicked** at the towel on the floor. Yep! He **dropped** things more frequently too. He **bent over** to **pick up** the towel and to **stretch** his back. That was stiffer too! He **stood up straight** and **rolled his shoulders forwards and backwards.** This usually relieved stress. He **sighed** loudly. *(Do you find change hard? Share some wisdom on how to adjust to life changes. What emotions might one have in making a move due to health issues or aging? What can you do to make it easier?)*

If he chose to **look** at this year through the eyes of his physical limitations, he would readily **wave** it good-bye! Why, he would even **open the door a**nd **push** it out! *(Let's push out all the not-so-good things that occurred this year and embrace the good memories. Share a good memory from this year.)*

But it had been a really good year as well. He connected with his grandson, discovered a new great-granddaughter, received a letter from his son, and won the king of the dining room for the Valentine's Day Luncheon at the Senior Center. He had **danced** with Dorothy that day! He would have **kissed** her, but she would have **punched** him if he had! But the thoughts were pleasant. He **breathed in and out slowly**, thinking about his favorite memories of the year.

He got to meet little Caitlin and grandson Jordan and his wife, Jenny. They had **hugged** and he **bounced** little Caitlin on his knee. She was only four months old! But she liked him! Jenny said so! He **smiled broadly** at the memories. *(Share about your* *grandchildren/greatgrandchildren. Have you had a reunion with someone you haven't seen in a long while? How did that make you feel? Who would you like to connect with?)*

He **reached his hands in the air** behind his back and **stretched** them over his head. Memories of his son filled his mind. He **swung his arms wildly** as he recalled the **roller coaster** rides they once loved together. So many fun things to think about. *(Tell me about some fun things you did with your family. Describe how you felt while doing them.)*

His son, Nathan, had married, then left for a war and never came back. He wasn't killed, thankfully, but he defaulted and stayed behind to help the locals. He **hung his head and shook it slowly.** He had lost communication just because of one bad statement. **He put his hand over his mouth** wishing he could have taken it back. *(Share some ways you might handle regrets. Have you ever made New Year's resolutions? Did you keep them? Do you make them now?)*

But all was well now! Nate had written. He was ok. And so is his family! Joe did a **little jig and put his heels and toes together** to celebrate. Too bad Margaret was gone. She was the love of his life! He **ran** to the kitchen to retrieve the towel that she had **embroidered.** Life was good back then. And he suddenly realized that he had let that year go, in the physical realm too, but never in his heart. *(What are some ways you can retain memories? Do you think what your heart cherishes ever goes away? Why or why not?)*

And so it would be with this one! He **put on his coat, ran a comb through his hair,** and **opened the door.** Might as well enjoy the fireworks! *(Talk about your New Year's celebrations. What do fireworks sound like? Feel like? Look like?)*

Charlotte Saben, ADC, AP-BC

Sharon and Sheila **giggled** like they did when they were kids. They **walked** and then **skipped** up the steps to the library. They knew their gaiety had to cease once inside. *(Do you enjoy going to the Library? Why or why not?)*

"Wait!" said Sheila. "I want to **take our picture** in front of this old library. It brings back memories and I want to keep them forever!" *(Do you think pictures help memories last forever?)*

"Don't count on that!" Sharon teased. "You can't even remember your grocery list anymore!"

They both **laughed** at the recalling of the scene of yesterday. They had **driven** Sharon's car to the store to buy strawberries and some other items Sheila desired. But Sharon had to **slam** on the brakes because a dog **ran** out in front of the car in the parking lot. She had missed it, thankfully, but **scolded** it like nobody's business! She **made faces** at it too. Every face she could think of! But the dog **trotted** off as if nothing had occurred. *(Have you ever hit or almost hit an animal?)*

And then when they began to **push** the shopping cart down the aisle, neither could remember what they had come for. Sharon, however, **reached i**nto her pocket and produced a list. "Coffee, Creamer, butter, bread, and butterscotch candy!" All things Sheila despised since she was a Vegan. Sheila put up her "dukes" as if **punching** Sharon, but did not. She didn't want to hurt her twin sister! But honestly! One would think by now that she would know how to properly eat! *(What is a Vegan? Do you think that is a good choice? Do you think Sharon's list was bad? Do you think diet affects our memories?) OR (Do you have or know any twins? Are you a twin? Share a story about that.)*

"So what do YOU need, Sister Dear?" Sharon had always liked to tease. Sheila **shrugged her shoulders** and **scratched her head**. For the life of her, she couldn't remember. And of course, she had NOT written it down! Sharon **looked up** as in disgust! She **rolled her eyes**. She **looked down** and **shook her head**. Sheila was stranger every time they got together. Sharon wouldn't admit that she had forgotten what Sheila came for as well.

Sheila **looked to the right and then to the left**. She **put her hands to her eyes** and **scanned** the aisle. Then she **marched** over to the meat counter and **pounded her fist**. "Such a waste of life!" she said. *(Do you think people should share their views publicly?)*

Sharon **pushed** her gently away and **pointed** her to the vegetables. That was more likely what she came for. Sheila **picked up** the bananas and looked them over.

"Nope!" she said. "Not organic!" She **tossed** a nearby apple into the air and **caught** it. "Too shiny. Means they put wax on it! They do that you know to make you buy the shinier ones! Don't ever do that!" She **stretched her arms over her head** and **sighed.** She **breathed in and out** several times to regain her composer.

Sharon used her **fingers, pinching them one at a time to her thumb**, to examine the strawberries. Her husband, Richard, really liked those. They were plump and red-ripe and looked very good. Then it hit her! THIS is what Sheila had wanted!

"Sheila! I think you wanted strawberries!" Sharon prompted her memory.

"Uh…I don't think I want ANYTHING in THIS store!" She said that rather loudly, so Sharon practically **ran** to the check-out to leave. Sheila didn't follow. Sharon found her seated at the door, **rolling her ankles, clicking her hills**, and **talking rapidly with her hands** to the young man re-stocking the produce. She was informing him of all the dangers of not being Vegan. *(Do you think her behavior should have embarrassed Sharon? Would you have been? Why/why not?)*

"I remembered when I found the RIGHT place to buy it!" The twins were back in the moment, **smiling broadly** into the phone. "Aren't selfies fun?"

"Yes, I wish we had phones capable of taking pictures back when we looked alike!" Sharon replied. *(Do you have a cell phone? Have you taken selfies on it?)*

"It would have been nice to have a phone at all! Or a camera that didn't require an army tote bag to transport! So, since you think we don't look alike, who looks better?" Sharon didn't answer Sheila's question. She **opened and closed her hands several times** and **opened the library door.** The "girls" did a little **jig** in the lobby and then put on their grown up, lady-like hats and entered the world of EVERYTHING! *(Why do you think they called the library the door to the world of Everything? What is your favorite book? Author? Story?)*

Charlotte Saben, ADC, AP-BC

Stan had been a stubborn little boy. You know, the active sort, always **running** and **jumping** and **climbing.** And he didn't like to listen. He often had **put his hands over his ears** when his mom tried to instruct him. *(Were you a naughty child? Were you or your children stubborn? How is that bad/good?)*

One day he **pedaled** his bike through the neighbor's garden! The neighbor **made a terrible face** and **shook his fist** at him. Then he **accentuated his vowels**! Stan **made several faces** when he tried to explain it all to his mother. *(What might he say "made" him do it?)*

It was only a week later when he **did a little jig** on his skateboard, with his **arms flapping up and down.** He was trying to be a dragon! He went **rolling** into the other neighbor's yard, but his skateboard **sailed** over the fence **hitting** the neighborhood tom cat who **howled** loudly. And that would start a series of unfortunate events! *(Have your neighbor's animals or kids ever bothered you? What did you do about it?)*

"Hey, YOU!" One of the neighbors was **stomping his feet** and **waving his arms**. "How many times we gotta tell you to watch out! It's time you learned a lesson!" He **marched** Stan up his front door and **knocked** loudly on it. Mom **opened** the door and **threw her hands in the air!** *(How would you have reacted if a neighbor marched your child home?)*

"Your kid needs a lesson! Maybe two or three! Maybe even a lifetime of them!" He was really mad!

Stan didn't like the sound of that. He imagined that Mr. Jones would have him **raking** leaves or **washing** cars or ALL the windows of his two-story house until he was ninety-nine! And maybe **walking** his crazy dog, Chainsaw, in the wee hours of the morning! Without a flashlight!

After Mr. Jones and Mom finished talking, Stan had a feeling it would be worse than that! He had seen Mom **nod** her head. Mr. Jones had **looked to the right and then to the left**. He **looked up and down**! Oh, no! What was he hoping to find? *(What kinds of chores did you have to do as a child? Did you like them?)*

Mr. Jones was known as the "piano man". It was partly because he **played the piano** at a local bar and at weddings. But he also "rescued" old ones, **refinished** and **tuned** them up! Stan imagined having to **scrub**, **scrape**, and refinish all those old ones he had seen in Mr. Jones' garage! He opened and closed his hands several times and moved each finger to the thumb; just warming them up for the inevitable! *(What is the strangest thing you have ever seen in a garage? Whose garage was it?)*

Yes, it turned out to be a punishment worse than he dreamed! He would definitely learn his lesson! One whole year of lessons! Piano lessons, that is! Mr. Jones wanted to turn Stan into the Piano Man! Stan **pouted**! He **punched the air with his fists.** This was way worse than **raking** leaves or **sweeping** the driveway! Why, if his friends found out, he'd be **laughed** at! *(Why do you think he felt like his friends would laugh at him? Did you or do you have friends that laugh at you? Why? What is the difference between laughing at someone and laughing with them?)*

Well, Stan lived through the entire experience! He **rolled his wrists in circles** and **tapped the air like he was playing a drum**. He was ninety now and still tickling those ivories, as they say! Stan discovered during that year, that he was actually good at **playing the piano**! He was good at music! He understood it and it understood him! He **clapped his hands** at the thought! *(Does music help you understand yourself? What song makes you feel happy? What other forms of "art" make you happy? What are you good at?)*

Mr. Jones had indeed made Stan into the Piano Man! Some of his friends thought that was weird. But he learned not to pay attention to that. He had indeed found something that made him **smile**; something that made his heart **beat** stronger! And here, eighty years and a fabulous career later, he had friends who really "got" him. He **wheeled** his wheelchair to the keyboard and **"hit"** it! *(How did you discover your career? Did you follow your heart?)*

Charlotte Saben, ADC, AP-BC

Alice **sipped** her smoothie and **licked her lips**. Why was it that Ruth and Gina were always late? She **looked to the right and then to the left**. No sign of them anywhere! She **looked up** at the second floor and saw Ruth **waving wildly**.

"Good grief!" Alice said. "They can't even find the right floor, much less the Juicy Juice!" Alice **waved** back, not so wildly, and **motioned** for them to come down right now! (*Have you ever gotten confused or lost trying to meet up with someone? How does that feel? How would you summon your friend?*)

Gina appeared at the top of the escalator and did her normal little **jig** before **stepping** on. Ruth **stretched her arms over her head** and **then bent to touch her toes**. She **glared** at Gina and promptly took the stairs! Ruth was glad the mall planners decided to leave them for those who prefer more exercise! She **rolled her neck** as she **descended the stairs**. (*Do you enjoy exercise? Why/why not?*)

As the three friends met up, Gina began her **full-fledged dance**, complete with **swinging hips**, **rolling ankles**, **tapping toes**, and **rolling shoulders**. Alice assumed Gina did this just to embarrass her. She **looked up and then down**. She **shook her head.** (*Do you have an embarrassing story to share? How does it make you feel when you're embarrassed?*)

"Hey! I told you that you need hearing aids! Can't you hear that wonderful band in the courtyard? They're right over there" she said, **pointing.** "Well, maybe it was over there!" She **pointed several directions**. Alice and Ruth just **rolled their eyes** and **made faces.** (*What kind of music do you enjoy? Do you like public dancing? Are/were you a dancer? Who did you dance with the most?*)

By this time, others were **watching**. Some joined in **the dance**, others **laughed.** Still others **put their hands on their hips** and **marched off.** Ruth and Gina did not see any band. Never mind! This mall is full of items **talking** to the ladies…**begging** them, pleading with them, to buy them and take them home. Perhaps all that sounds like music to Gina's ears! (*Can you imagine items talking to you? Have you ever used the expression: "It was just calling out to me!"?*)

The trio **walked** down the hall to the left.

"Diamonds! Truly a girl's best friend! Just too bad I'm not a girl anymore!" Gina always had something clever to say. She **opened and closed her hands several times.** She **smiled** as she looked at the ring on her finger. Boyd had given that to her some fifty years ago now. She **hugged herself** the way she knew he would have. *(Did someone special ever give you a diamond? Did you give someone a diamond? What is your favorite gem? What is your birthstone?)*

Gina hadn't noticed that Ruth and Alice had **walked** away. They didn't notice she wasn't with them either. They had been so busy **chatting**, and she, so busy reminiscing and **staring** at diamonds, that they had become separated.

For a moment, Gina was scared. She **put her hands to her forehead and peered into the crowd.** They just disappeared! Gone! Just like that! Gina was concerned since she had ridden with Ruth. But, she decided to make the best of it until she figured something out. *(What would you do if you became separated from the person you rode somewhere with?)*

There was a large lady dress shop! Just her size! She liked to try on clothes. She **pulled** the pants on and **wiggled her bottom** just a bit. Nice fit! She **raised her arms** to try on the blouse but got her elbow stuck in the sleeve! She **moved her elbow in circles** until it worked its way back into the sleeve! No wonder!She had it on backwards!*(Have you ever accidentally worn clothes backwards or inside-out? Have you gone to a backwards party? Ever had a mishap while trying on clothing in a store?)*

Her next stop was the pet store! She knew she should just look from the outside, but…the next thing she knew she was **petting** a puppy and **giving kisses** to a myna bird who was **whispering** in her ear.Too much temptation in there! She **opened the door** widely and **walked** out. *(Do you like animals? What is your favorite? Do you remember your first pet? Describe it to us.)*

Gina stopped at the candy store to **taste** the fudge. Yummy! And then she went to the shoe store to **try on** some slippers. She **clicked her toes and then her heels together** to make sure the fit was right. She didn't escape that store without **carrying several bundles!** *(Describe your favorite shoe, shirt or outfit.)*

Gina ended up in the most amazing room of all! Room, yes. Store, no. It was full of children of all ages. It was so noisy that she was glad she had not worn her hearing aids, a fact that Ruth and Alice must never know. She **put her hands over her ears** briefly and then decided to brave the noise. She **put in the token** a young man had given her, **pulled back** on the "throttle" and let the action begin. The ball **bounced** from one side to the other while Gina frantically **pushed** and **pulled** at the knobs **swatting** at the ball. She used up three balls in less than two minutes! That must be a pinball record! She **pulled her shoulders back** and

Charlotte Saben, ADC, AP-BC

patted her back. She was very proud! An older gentleman **shook her hand** and then **shook his head**. He **turned** away, not wanting her to see him **laugh.** *(Have you ever played pinball? Do you like arcade games? Video games? Which ones?)*

Suddenly Gina felt her purse **shaking**! What was it? She held back the scream trying to escape. Another young man said, "Lady, I think your cell phone is **ringing!"** Gina felt silly. She **reached** in her purse and **pulled out** the ringing and **vibrating** phone.

"Hello."

"Where ARE you?" It was Alice. Always proper Alice!

"I'm in pinball heaven. I just set a record!"

"That's GAME HAVEN, Ma'am" a young girl replied.

After **handing** the phone to the girl to give directions, Gina **took a deep breath**. Perhaps Ruth and Alice had deserted her on purpose! Maybe she had really embarrassed them with her **dancing**. No matter. She had had a wonderful adventure!

And suddenly, the room turned to **dancing**. Gina found herself **sliding** across the floor with a most handsome teen! Yes, she had had the best day of all.

Alice and Ruth could only **stare** and **drop their jaws**! *(Do you relate well to younger people? Do you think there is a generation gap? Why/why not?)*

Marcia **loved** the color green. *(hug yourself)* *(What is your favorite color and what does it remind you of?)* It reminded her of things that **grow. (Make motions like sprouts coming up from the ground with both fingers and hands, or with exaggerated arm motions, etc.)** She was a gardener at heart and always would be. *(Do you like gardening? What have you grown in the past?)*

She **pulled** the weeds from the garden bed and **threw** them into the trash bin. **(This could become a game of tossing a ball, balloon, paper, etc. into a trash can or just making the tossing motions.)** She **kicked** at a rock that tried to make her stumble. She **walked** through the gate of the larger garden, **opening** it wide.

She **took a deep breath**. She **breathed in and out** several times, taking in the smell of the "clean" dirt and vegetables. She loved that smell! *(Describe the smell of "clean dirt". Do you like that smell? What garden smells do you like?)* **(At this point, introduce things to smell…dirt, onions or onion flakes, spices, etc.)**

She **looked to the right and then to the left.** No signs of any bunnies or other critters that liked to **eat** in her garden. She **looked up and then down**. No signs of foul weather. But, wait! What is that? She **bent down** to examine the hole. Oh No! She **made a face of disgust!** She **made several other faces** as well. She **rolled her neck** and **rolled her eyes**. She **scratched** her head. She would think of something! It looked like a gopher might be trying to make his home in this garden! *(Have you ever had to fight with gophers or other critters in your yard? What methods did you use to get them out?)*

Marcia **stomped** out of the garden and into the garage. She **reached** up and **unhooked** a large hose from the wall and **dragged** it to the garden area where she **twisted** the end onto the facet. She **pushed** the hose down into the hole, making sure it was securely positioned. By now she had discovered the other hole, confirming indeed that it was a gopher. She **turned on** the water! She hoped that Mr. Gopher was home.

She **held** the hose tightly, **opening and closing her fingers** around it.

Suddenly, she **yelled** excitedly and did a little **jig.** There he was! **Running** out the other hole as fast as he could!

She hoped he got the message! Stay out of the garden!!! Soon Marcia knew that the gopher would not return. The neighborhood tom cat spotted him and **gave chase!**

 Charlotte Saben, ADC, AP-BC

Marcia did a **side-step dance** and **cheered, waving her arms** rather wildly. She wasn't sure who she was rooting for, but this was the most excitement she'd seen all week!

Marcia didn't find out what happened to the gopher. She didn't really want to know who won that race. The tom cat seemed to return with a **smile** on his face, however. And she never saw that gopher again! *(Do you think the cat caught the gopher? How would you feel about that?)*

Ed had never been to the gym before and he didn't want to go today! He **pouted** and **made a fist** and **shook it.** Then he **opened and closed his hands** several times. They didn't want to go either! They said so by the popping sound they made. He **moved each finger individually to the thumb** to loosen them up, but they made noise then as well. No matter! Ruth was NOT going to budge about this! *(Have you had to do something you didn't want to just to please someone?)*

He hadn't really meant to agree to this! Ruth caught him **licking** the cake she had made for the church bake sale! That's all! He'd used his **fingers!** *(Lick fingers)* Such punishment didn't fit the crime! He **kicked** at the car door and **dropped** his keys! He **bent over** to get them and suddenly had an idea! He **looked up and then down**. He **looked to the right** and **then to the left**. There wasn't anyone watching! *(Did you ever lick frosting off a cake? What did it taste like? Feel like? Smell like? Did you get caught? What would you do if someone licked your cake?)*

He pretended to **slip**, ending up **sitting** on the front lawn **twirling his ankles** in circles and **making faces!** He **waved his arms wildly** as if he needed an ambulance! He **moaned** and **accentuated his vowels!** *(Have you ever pretended to be hurt or sick to get out of something? What are some other ways to get out of it?)*

Ruth came **running** out of the house!

"Mercy me!" she said. "How in tarnation did you end up here? All I asked you to do was **get in the car** to go to the gy…Oh! I get it!" *(Would you have suspected your friend or spouse? Why or why not?)*

She **walked** over to the car and opened the door.

"I guess I'll just go without you!" she said. "If you can't **get up**, just **call** George next door on your cell phone in your pocket and he'll come **lift** you up! Bye!" She **climbed** into the driver's seat, having **picked up** the keys Ed had **dropped** again in his "fall".

She **turned the ignition with her wrist**. The engine hummed. She **shut the door.**

She **put the car in gear**. She **honked** the horn! *(What do you think it sounded like? Was it loud? Did it vibrate?)*

"Hey! Wait just a minute!" Ed declared. "You can't drive my prized possession! That's my **baby!**" (***Cuddle your arms to your chest like you're holding a baby.***)

He **jumped up** and **pulled open** the door. *(Did you ever have a special car? How did you protect it? Did you ban anyone else from driving it? What was your favorite possession?)*

"My! How fast your ankle healed!" Ruth said with a **grin**. "Now let's go to the gym! Get **moving** before I **march** back in the house and get your checkbook to **sign** you up for a whole year of classes!"

Ed **moved his arms up and down** as if he had barbells. He **flexed his muscle**, but Ruth wasn't impressed! He **moved his arms in circles**, but she just **tossed** him the keys! Ed **stretched his arms in the air** like he was surrendering to a policeman! And then he **caught** the keys!

"Get in!" she said. The engine continued to hum…

(Have you ever been to a gym? What are some of the classes they might offer? What are some exercises they might do?) (***Move arms like swimming, rowing, and move legs like on a treadmill, etc.***)

Annie **wrapped** the scarf around her neck and **turned her head from side to side**. She was both excited and nervous. She was mad at Debbie for backing out of this trip; and she was glad she was going it alone. She **sighed** and **made a face**. She hadn't realized she had this in her. She felt brave and scared at the same time. She **kicked** at a leaf that tried to attach itself to her luggage. She **dragged** the suitcase through the line and **lifted** it onto the scale. *(Have you ever traveled abroad? Were you alone? Who was with you? Where did you go? Why?)*

Ticket in hand, she **walked** to the customs line. She **pulled** her passport out of her bag and **waved** it in the air. She would be very careful with this! She **hugged** it to her heart and **gave herself a hug**. This would be a very special adventure! *(Do you like to travel by plane? Why or why not? What other modes of travel have you experienced?)*

The plane was the biggest she had ever been on! She **climbed** the stairs leading to the entrance ramp carefully. She didn't want to **trip**. Her seat was a middle one! Just her luck! Oh, well. She could meet new people and **chat** like best friends! *(Are you shy or outgoing? Do you like to meet strangers?)*

Annie tried to **converse** with the man in the window seat, but he fell asleep immediately and began to **snore**. Oh, rats! The lady in the aisle seat was friendly enough but **chattered** on in a language foreign to Annie. She **nodded** and **smiled.** *(Have you tried to talk to someone who did not speak your language? How did that feel? Have you been in a foreign country and unable to speak the language?)*

Annie **pulled** out her book and began to **read**. It seemed only moments that she felt the plane **descend.** *(Make motions with arms like a plane descending: raising and swooping motions)* The Captain made announcements in English and some language she assumed was Japanese, since the airline was. She **shivered** a bit because this was her first time in a foreign country. And she was only half-way to her destination. *(What do you do to pass time while traveling?)*

She **raised her arms** in the air and **swayed like a tree**. No one seemed to notice and if they did they would probably just think "silly American!" She **bent down** to **stretch her back**. The "moment" of travel had really been ten hours! She **rolled her ankles around** and **tapped her toes**. She wasn't sure if she had been lost in her book or sound **asleep** dreaming, but the time had **flown** by. She didn't have to go through Customs at least at this lay-over! *(Do long trips get you down or do you enjoy them? Share about a trip you have taken.)*

The next leg of her journey would begin in five hours. She **pulled out** her IPad and **plugged** it into the outlet. She had purchased the appropriate adapter at least! She began **typing furiously**. She had so much to put in her diary already! She **watched** the other planes land and take off. She **opened and closed her hands** several times; They were a little stiff due to her habit of **typing** too long! She **shook her hands,** then **wandered** into a store to **pick up** a souvenir or two. **Exchanging** American money for Japanese was interesting. She **pushed the buttons** on the machine and **hoped** she did it right. *(Have you ever exchanged money in a strange machine? Were you apprehensive? Do the new machines and banking techniques bother you?)*

She **approached** the food kiosk and **pointed** to the picture on the menu. The waiter **nodded** and began to **cook** it immediately. She wasn't completely sure what it was, but she was hungry and would **eat** just about anything! *(What's the strangest thing you have eaten? Are you adventurous with food?)*

She **ate** and **drank** slowly, **sipping** her tea delicately. Manners were important here, it was obvious. She **breathed deeply** several times and **closed her eyes**. *(Do you think manner should be important? Is our society lacking in manners? How do you think our culture could be influenced?)*

She **tried to imagine** what lie ahead for her and what adventures she might face. She **rolled her neck** around and allowed her mind to **wander.** She was off on a very exciting adventure indeed! *(Where do you wish you had gone? What would you still like to see?)* **(At this point, you can share post cards or travel videos on UTube or some other site. OR hand out artifacts or souvenirs from another country to feel and spices to smell and teas, coffee to taste etc.)**

It had been a long trip and Annie **yawned**. She **stretched her arms in the air** and **arched her back**. She **rolled her ankles around** and **raised first her heels and then her toes.** She would be meeting someone new shortly. Her daughter, Jill, had arranged for an escort through, or around, the Customs system and then to meet up with her outside the airport. Security was different here. Some things tighter; some looser. She had never been met at an airport before by a sign with her name on it! **Seeing** that kind of made her feel important! *(Would that make you feel important? What does make you feel important?)*

She **followed** the young ladies down the long hallway, **walking slowly** and carefully while **dragging** her **rolling** suitcase. *(**Either do a walking motion with feet or a sweeping, "following" motion with hands for "followed" and "rolling" motions with hands.)*** They seemed nice, but Annie had thought they would be more fluent in English. They **gestured** with their hands which way to go. She **nodded.** They **smiled.** They **hurried** past long lines and straight to a coffee kiosk! Coffee is everywhere! Good thing she **loved** it! She **reached** into her wallet to buy all of them a treat, but realized her money was now American and Japanese. This was neither. *(Have you ever traveled to a foreign country? What did you find difficult to adjust to? Was it a military, business, or pleasure trip?)* *(**If no one has, share a short travel video at the end of the group session and proceed with discussion following.)***

Annie **opened and closed her hands several times**, feeling a little awkward. The ladies were **texting** on their phones and then **chatting** in an unfamiliar tongue. They seemed a little stressed. One **took several long deep breaths** and then **looked to the right and to the left**. She **pointed** and **laughed!**

There, in the sweltering heat, **walking rapidly** was her daughter, Jill! They **embraced.** *(**Hug yourself several times, crossing opposite arms each time.)*** All the ladies **looked** at each other, **made funny faces** and **laughed**. Apparently, Jill had used some words incorrectly, having made a sentence hilarious! But laughter is the same in any language! Jill treated them all to coffee. As Annie **sipped** her coffee, she **relaxed**. She **rolled her neck around** and **bent her head from side to side**. She had been able to **sleep** on the plane, but it wasn't comfortable at all! *(Have you used a foreign word improperly? What was the outcome? What might be an outcome?) OR (Do you like to travel? Sleep on a plane?)*

Annie was amazed to see big city buses sharing the same streets as horse-drawn taxis and becaks, and **bicycles!** *(**Make motions like you are driving a horse buggy and bicycling)*** Every parking lot they passed made her **stare in awe,** because there were 100 motorcycles

Charlotte Saben, ADC, AP-BC

to one truck or van! Quite different from her Phoenix city lots she was used to. *(Make motions like you are driving a truck; you can even have them honk!) (Also a good time to show travel videos or pictures of countries where this is the norm—Asian countries like Indonesia, Thailand, etc.)* *(Have you driven in a foreign country? Ridden in a taxi pulled by an animal? What might it sound like? Smell like? Look like?)* *(What is a becak? What country might she be in?)* *(A good opportunity if you have Internet to do a research project on this.)*

Every bit of this trip would be amazing! The twenty hours of **flying** seemed like only a few now that she was here! And boarding a train for another six seemed fine. *(Residents can make train sounds.)* She **swayed** back and forth both on her feet and in her seat as the train **chugged** across the landscape. *(Tell us about traveling on a train. Does anyone collect trains? Been an Engineer or Brakeman? Or worked on the Railroad?)* *(Can discuss about trains being part of the pioneer westward movement, etc. Any history on trains would fit here.)*

Annie **pedaled** many miles in the following week. She **walked,** she **ran,** she **jogged** across amazing country. She **climbed** hills, **ran up** and down **stairs** of ancient temples and **swatted** at flies in open street markets. She **smelled** *(breathe in)* the fresh gardens and stinky sheep. *(Hold noses.)* She **dodged** motorcycles while crossing streets without the benefit of traffic lights. She even **rode** behind a stranger on a motorcycle across a bamboo bridge, **hanging on** for dear life! She never knew she was so brave! *(Do you think that was brave or crazy?)* *(What is something that has made you feel brave?)*

Jill misses Annie and **calls** when she can. And Annie misses Jill, and the amazing country she discovered. She **counts** the days until her next opportunity to find that it's a small world after all.

(Might lead singing of "It's A Small World" or listen to it online, or show a Disneyland clip.) (This story could lead to all sorts of discussions about travel, the differences and similarities of countries, etc.)

Ginny and Jessie loved being together like most grandmas and granddaughters. The first thing they always did was **wave** their special "princess" **wave** and **open and close their hands several times.** They weren't quite sure what benefit that had, but it made them both **laugh.** They shared an extra-special bond because they both loved baking more than almost anything.

Perhaps it all started when Jessie was only three and started helping "Gama Gin-Gin" **frost** her famous Holiday cupcakes and cookies. Sweet breads and pies, fruit cakes and candies became famous too. There seemed to be nothing Ginny couldn't bake or make. And Ginny gave away as many as she sold, but the money always went to the homeless shelter or the rescue mission anyway. Everybody deserves a happy Holiday Ginny thought. Jessie **smiled** knowing what her grandmother was thinking. Even though she was a teenager now, she still loved doing this wonderful adventure together. *(What memories do you have of doing things with your children? Grandchildren?)* ***(You can make motions like stirring, opening oven, using a mixer, etc.)***

Ginny **opened the refrigerator** and **plopped** the dough on the counter. She made a **puff of flour rise** as the dough hit it squarely in the center. Ginny was a pro! Jessie began **rolling the dough** as quickly as she could. She **bent down** to make sure the oven was on. Occasionally Gama Gin-Gin (as she still affectionately called her) forgot to **flip the knob** to "on". Gama Gin-Gin **rolled her eyes** and then **her neck**, pretending to have a cramp. She **looked down** at the oven door. The light was on. The oven was not. Ginny **looked up** and **made a face**, mostly at herself. *(Did you ever forget to turn on the oven? Crockpot? Coffee pot?)*

Jessie **patted the dough** as she **dipped** the cookie cutters in the flour. A reindeer. A Christmas tree. A dreidel. Ginny didn't like leaving anyone out. Jessie wondered where she had found that cookie cutter.

"There's a menorah as well. Leave it Gin-Gin!" Ginny **stretched her arms over her head** and said something in Romanian. Then she **swung her arms wildly and swatted a wayward fly**. Such creatures were NOT allowed in Ginny's kitchen!

Ginny **squeezed** the icing onto the cupcake with the ease of an expert. Then she **sprinkled** "sparkles" all over them. So pretty! She **moved each finger to her thumb and back twice.** Jessie noticed she didn't move quite as quickly as before. No matter; Jessie would make up for it. She felt energized just by being with her grandmother. *(Did you like spending time with your grandmother/grandfather? What did you do together?)*

Charlotte Saben, ADC, AP-BC

Jessie **bent down** again, this time **bending her knees**, to put the cookie sheets in the oven. She **reached** in quickly to center them. She **stepped back** and **wiped her brow**. Baking was hot work, even with snow on the ground outside!

Speaking of snow, Jessie's brother, Jeremy was outside **shoveling** it! He actually liked doing that! Jessie didn't understand that, but Jeremy didn't understand her love of hot stoves either! She **shook her head** at the thought! *(Did you like shoveling snow?)*

Jessie **walked** to the door to let Jeremy in. She gave him a little **punch** on the shoulder. He **pushed** her back. Gama Gin-Gin would have intervened, but she knew it was all in fun. Besides, she had a cup of hot chocolate waiting for him. She **poured** some cream on it to cool it down just a smidgen. Jeremy **sat down** and **kicked** his feet towards the fireplace. *(Do you like hot chocolate? What do you like to drink when it's cold outside?)*

He knew it was he who should get up and **stoke the fire** a bit. But he was tired. It was also he who was cold. The ladies were **fanning** themselves over the open refrigerator door while the cookies baked. Ginny had already baked four dozen cupcakes, six sweet breads, three pumpkin pies (from scratch, no less) and a couple dozen persimmon cookies! All before the kids arrived at 10 AM! Jeremy **stomped** the snow from his boots and **got up** to **mop** up the mess. He knew he should have done the **stomping** at the door before **stepping** into the house. Since he was up, he might as well, **stoke** AND **mop**…and get some more hot chocolate! *(Did you bake? What did you bake? Did you like to cook? What is your specialty?)*

Jessie **wiped down the counter** and **washed** the cookie sheets. Ginny was **licking** the remains of the frosting off the spatula. She was very careful to be completely finished **frosting** before **licking**…but she sure did enjoy that routine. She was a kid at heart!

Jeremy **carried** the boxes of goodies to the car. Jessie would **drive.** She had her license and Ginny didn't love driving any more. Jessie **smiled** remembering last year when she was too young to drive. Gama Gin-Gin had **swerved** to miss a squirrel and then had to **slam on her brakes** to avoid a **run**-away dog. One of the cakes slid off the seat and landed right in Jessie's lap! Avoiding that dog became an even bigger issue when Jessie got out of the car! *(Have you ever hit or almost hit an animal with your car? How did you feel?)*

But this year would be different. Jessie knew how to drive in the snow, safely avoid animals and **bee-bop to music** all at the same time. Ginny bee-bopped along too, much to Jeremy's surprise. He was in the back seat, **holding onto the goodies**, and **reciting his prayers under his breath!** He **took some deep breaths, in and out.** He **closed his eyes and imagined** himself back in the cozy home of Gama Gin-Gin, safely **sleeping** on the sofa! *(Were you ever scared enough to pray while someone was driving?)*

"Hey, YOU!" Jeremy **jumped** and **sat up straight**! "Come help with those boxes, Sleepyhead!"

"I…I wasn't sleeping. I was pray---." Maybe it wasn't such a good idea to reveal his prayer time. Jessie might really **punch** for that!

The rescue mission and homeless shelter both praised them all for the delivery. The men, women, and children in both places **clapped** and **cheered**. Jeremy decided to join in when they invited them to all **sing** along. "Deck the Halls…Jingle Bells…"

Jeremy did a little **dance** for them as well. He **chomped** down on a cookie as he **waved** goodbye, **leaping** into the car as Jessie **steered** away. *(Do you like caroling? Singing Holiday songs? What celebrations do you do? Do you have special traditions to share?)*

"Happy Holidays! Merry Christmas! Happy Hanukkah! Happy Kwanzaa! We just want to celebrate people! God Bless Us Everyone!"

Charlotte Saben, ADC, AP-BC

Cliff **sat up straight**. He **stretched his arms over his head** and **yawned** widely. Today would be filled with adventure. He **rubbed his upper arms** with his hands. He **rubbed his hand togethe**r and **opened and closed them** several times. Yes, indeed! This day was like no other! *(Do you anticipate an adventurous day?)*

His wife, Barbara **walked** into the room **dragging** a suitcase. She **lifted** it up onto the bed next to Cliff. *(Who packed your suitcase? Did you pack everyone else's?)*

"There!" She said. "That ought to get you through the week!" Cliff **looked to the left and then to the right**. Barbara did the same. "Whatcha looking for now?" she asked.

"Nothing" he said as he **looked down and then up** and did it again. Barbara **shook her head** and **stomped** out of the room. It wasn't that she was angry. She was excited for Cliff. It was just that his way of handling nervousness made her nervous! Cliff would be **flying** today; his very first time on a commercial plane. The last time he was on any plane was in the military and his memories weren't so kind. Sometimes he had awakened with bad dreams. But that had not happened in several years now. She couldn't help but worry, though. That was her job as his wife. He would never admit to worrying! He just **tapped his fingers** and **rolled his ankles repeatedly** lately. She knew the sign. She **made a face**. *(Have you ever flown on a commercial jet? Tell us about it. Were you nervous? Why or why not. OR Would anyone like to share about military service? Was anyone a pilot? Airplane mechanic?)*

"Did you pack my lucky shorts?" Cliff inquired. He **bent down** to **pull on** his bright green socks, which he deemed lucky as well. *(Do you have lucky clothing? Charms? Numbers?)*

"Of course, Dear!"

"I think you should **unpack** those and put them in the carry-on! That way I'll be sure the plane won't go down!" He **made flying motions with his arms** and then **flapped them** like a panicked bird. Barbara was in the other room and wouldn't comment. It was another way to relieve his stress. *(What relieves your stress?)*

He truly wanted to take this trip to see his daughter, Melanie. He hadn't seen her in close to twenty years! The reasons **raced** through his mind and **his feet tapped to the rhythm**. Barbara heard the commotions. She had also heard the comment.

"If those silly shorts can keep the plane air-born then you should auction them to the highest bidder once you get home!" She **laughed** a nervous laugh. She didn't particularly enjoy air travel, though she had done plenty in her 70 plus years. Her children, too, were scattered all across the nation. *(Where does your family live? OR What are some other ways of travel that you have experienced?)*

Cliff **danced** his way into the room and **hugged** Barbara. It had been many years now since she **danced** her way into his heart! She had filled a lonely void that his own mistakes had created. She helped him forgive himself. He **took a deep breath**. He **breathed in and out several times** and **rolled his neck around both directions.** He **kissed** her tenderly on her cheek. He wished she could go with him at least for moral support. But this was something he needed to do alone. *(Who has helped you forgive yourself?)*

Barbara had been the catalyst between Melanie and Cliff. He **smiled** at the thought. Barbara really loved him and certainly knew how to be a diplomat. He **ate** his breakfast quickly. *(What is your favorite breakfast food? Can you eat it quickly?)*

He heard the shuttle **drive** up. The driver **knocked** on the door lightly, **picked up** the suitcase and practically **ran** to the van. The two lovers **embraced** and then **waved** goodbye. Cliff knew his adventure would be a great one. And he would look forward to Barbara's **smile** upon his return. Now his thoughts drifted to memories of Melanie so very long ago. (*share fond memories of your children or your own childhood. OR share a story about a trip you took.)*

Charlotte Saben, ADC, AP-BC

Margaret **reached** up and **plucked** the citrus from the tree. *(What kind of citrus do you like best? What does the smell make you think of? The taste?)*

She **kicked** at the clod of dirt she felt on her feet. She **rolled her ankles** and **tapped her heels together and then her toes.**

"GRrrr! Arf! Arf!" Sassy, the Chihuahua wasn't about to arise just yet. Margaret **rolled her neck around** and then **made a face**. She was still in bed! She had been dreaming!

She sat up quickly then bent over slowly to **put her feet in her slippers**. *(What would your slippers look like? Feel like? Have you ever had an animal sleep in your bed?)*

She **licked her lips** anticipating that orange she had just **picked** in her dream! She hoped she had one in the kitchen. She didn't have an orange tree any more. She missed her small orchard back home. Home. The physical location of "home" had changed several times over Margaret's lifetime. *(How many different places have you lived in? Which was your favorite? What sounds, smells, sights to you recall most vividly?)*

She missed the **hikes** in the hills of Kentucky. She missed **riding her horse** on the ranch in Texas. She missed **watering** the small citrus grove she had in Florida. She missed the **bicycling** she and David had done in Portland, Oregon. She **breathed in deeply**. In and out. **In and out**. It gave her a refreshed mind with which to cherish her memories.

Now here she was in the desert of Arizona. David and she had come here on vacation to **golf**, **swim**, **climb**, and **explore**. She didn't like to **climb** as much as he did, but she enjoyed watching the birds along the way. ***(Make motions like you have binoculars and move head from side to side and up and down)*** *(What kind of exploring have you done? Did you enjoy it? What did you enjoy on vacations?)*

They never intended to stay here. But plans change. And here she is, alone in yet a different state. At least she has one niece nearby. She comes to visit and they **bake cookies** together. ***(Make motions like rolling out dough, and cutting out cookies, open and shut the oven, etc.)*** They **sing** a lot too. And Cassie **plays the piano** for Margaret. That is always a pleasure, since Margaret was the one who taught her to play! *(Let's sing a few of your favorite songs! Did you ever play an instrument? Teach anyone else to play?)*

Cassie liked to think that she could interpret dreams too! That gave Margaret a good **laugh**, although she had to admit that sometimes Cassie seemed to get to the bottom of Margaret's feelings through explaining her dreams. Margaret had never been much for paranormal type things and dream interpretation had seemed a lot like that. *(Do you remember any dreams* *you've had? Any that repeated themselves? Do you think there might be underlying meaning to them?)*

Margaret couldn't help but wonder what Cassie would say about that big orange she dreamed about and couldn't get out of her head? She remembered a discussion that they had about colors of dreams…. Ah yes…Orange…what did that mean again? *(At this point, if you have any info on color or dream interpretation, you might share it.)*

By now Sassy was **yipping loudly** and **clawing** at the door. And Cleo the Siamese cat was **meowing** in her own special way. *(Show me how Cleo might look when she meowed. What pets did you have to wake up to?)* Time to **walk** into the kitchen, let Sassy out the door, and put the coffee pot on. She **looked up at the sky** as she **opened the door**. Nice day! Good feel to the air. She **opened and closed her hands several times**. They were not as stiff as usual. Going to be a nice day! She **glanced** *(roll eyes)* at the note on the fridge. Today was Sunday! Cassie would be coming! It was definitely going to be a good day! She **did a little dance step** and **clapped her hands**. She even **gave herself a hug** and **said out loud, "Yes, it's a very nice day, indeed!"**

She watched it go up. She watched it come down. She watched it go up and she watched it come down. She watched it go…halfway up and then all the way! She watched as it came down halfway and then all the way to the floor**! *(At this point, have the residents move their arms up in the air above their heads and then down as far as you want them to go including all the way to the floor if possible! They should move the arms only halfway up and down at the appropriate cues. They could move their heads up and down in addition or as an alternate.)***

And then the inside disappeared completely! She knew that it must have gone to the basement this time! She wasn't sure she wanted to ride in that thing where everyone could see her. Even worse, she would have to see everything as she ascended. All that was scary! Besides the line was getting longer and longer for the brand-new elevator in this fancy store! It had been **the talk** of the town for several months. **(*Make chatty movements with fingers or mouths.*)** This is a top-of-the-line "open" windows-all-around elevator going from the third floor all the way to the basement parking lot! *(Have you seen a new invention or fancy elevator that was intimidating?)*

She **bent down** and **picked up** the five shopping bags, **slinging** one of them over her shoulder along with her purse. She would take the escalator. At least they still had that choice! As Lynda **walked** to the escalator, she **sighed deeply**. Then she **took a deep breath**! She **looked up** at the metal staircase that was completely still. She **looked down** at the floor. The sign was huge! "Escalator temporarily out of order…try our new elevator! Sorry for the inconvenience!" She **dropped** her bags and **made a face**. She felt like **crying**! Maybe they were just trying to promote that new monstrosity! She **looked to the left and then to the right**.She saw the old stairway, full of people just like herself. *(Did you prefer the elevator, escalator, or stairs? Why?)*

She **stretched her arms out as if she could fly**. She truly wished she could. She **pumped her arms** up and down with the bags hanging helplessly attached only by flimsy handles. She tried to imagine herself **rising** above the crowd. But, alas! She would take those stairs! After all, her doctor had just told her she needed more exercise! He had suggested going to a gym three times a week. Lynda figured that if carrying these bags up the flight of stairs wasn't good enough exercise, then the doctor could go to the gym himself! She practically **stomped** over to the stairs and **marched** up them as fast as she could! *(What is your favorite form of exercise? At a gym?)*

She loved the baby section! It had been some time since she **rocked** a baby or **patted** one on the back. She **walked** to the canopy crib and **moved the side rail up and down.** It was a new kind with a foot release. She **pressed her feet up and down** on the lever. It was kind of fun. She felt like a naughty kid in the candy store! *(Do you like children? How many grandchildren/children/nieces/nephews/etc. do you have? Any babies?)*

Next she tried the strollers. She **pushed one back and forth** across the aisle. She **bent** to unlatch the handlebars and **folded** it up just as the clerk **tapped her foot**. "May I help you, Ma'am?" Lynda could tell the clerk was a bit agitated. She **pointed** to the sign. "Please do not play with the products." *(Have you ever done something daring or silly or bad in a store as an adult?)*

"Oops!" Lynda **put her hand to her mouth**. "I'm sorry." Lynda didn't say anything else because she knew she intended to play some more!

She casually **crisscrossed** her way down the aisle out of sight of the clerk. She **picked up** a rattle and began to **shake** it. Surely that wouldn't be enough to alarm the clerk! She **pushed** the button on the "Light-up Daisy Dog" expecting only lights. Instead, the dog began to **bark** and **bounce up and down** in the package! Lynda **ran** down the aisle and **hunched her shoulders** to try to hide. The clerk **kicked** at a toy on the floor, **put her hands on her hips and twisted from side to side**. She did not see Lynda! Hooray! *(Do you think it was okay for Lynda to do this? Why or why not?)*

Lynda suddenly remembered that she had left her bags on the floor beside the crib! Oh, no! She would have to find a way to get them! She **rolled her ankles in circles** to make sure her shoes wouldn't squeak. **She touched her toes together and then her heels** to limber up before her daring deed! She was ready!!! *(What would you have done?)*

With a big **heave**, Lynda **knocked** over an entire rack of diapers! While the clerk was **rushing** to the commotion, Lynda **raced** to the crib, **grabbed** her packages and **ran down** the stairs! *(If you had seen Lynda's actions, would you have told on her? Why or why not?)*

She heard the call as she descended:

"Security please! To the third floor stat!" and "Stockers to third floor on the double!"

Lynda knew she was very wrong. She **hung her head**. But it had been years since she had done such daring deeds! Not since her granddaughter and she had accidentally **bumped** into the display of hats at the mall, had she had such a **laugh**! *(What should she do? Would you go home or confess? Why might she have done such things?)*

Charlotte Saben, ADC, AP-BC

He **stomped** heartily on the mat. He **shook** his feet, first one and then the other. The snow scattered over the porch and onto the walls of the house. He **stepped** into the warm, cozy living room where a fire was blazing, (*Does it feel better to be in the snow or in the warm house? Which did you prefer when you were younger?*)

He had just been outside **throwing** snowballs at his grandchildren, *(you can do not only the throwing exercise, but also a rolling or squishing motion as if making a snowball*), but he looked like he had gotten the worse end of the event. He **took off his hat** and **shook his head**, **rolling his neck** from side to side. He **looked to the left**. He **looked to the right.** He **looked up and down.** He **rolled his shoulders forward and backwards**.

"Wow! Those kids have a good aim!" He thought it aloud, but no one heard him. *(Have you ever had a snowball fight with your grandchildren? Children? Who won? How did the snow feel?) (What other games did you or do you play with others?)*

He **flung** his coat off his shoulders and onto the rack. He **stretched his arms out and over his head, making circles** as he did. He wondered what it would be like to be a forest animal out in this snow. (*What kinds of animals might be out in the snow? What sounds would they make? What would they eat? What animals have you seen in the wild in the winter?*)

He sat down to a nice cup of coffee. He **breathed in and out deeply.** It smelled so good to him! (*What smells good to you? Do you like coffee? Tell me what smells you like? What drinks do you like?*)

He **pulled** his gloves off and shook his fingers. He **made a fist and then relaxed** his hands, over and over again. He hadn't realized they were a bit numb. He **shook his wrists** and **moved his fingers to his thumb.** He **sipped** his coffee and **blew** on it gently. He **made some faces** just to unfreeze his cheeks!

He knew he only had a few moments before the children would **walk** in. He **got up** *(if unable to stand, have them make walking motions or motions like wheeling in a wheelchair)* and **poked** at the fire in the fireplace and **kicked** at a log on the hearth. He **bent down** to tie his bootlace. He **touched his toes** and **then his knees**. Everything seemed to be normal after that workout!

He **pushed himself up** and **stretched** his back. He heard a **knock** at the door. Must be the grandkids! He **marched** to the door and **opened** it wide. *(Tell me about your grandchildren.)*

In **jumped** a squirrel! It **hopped** up on the table. He **bounced** off the wall. The grandpa **shut** the door and then **reopened** it quickly as the squirrel **leaped** outside again. He spotted a bear behind the tree and **opened his mouth** to yell.

He heard **a giggle** and then **a laugh**! He noticed that the bear was really small and had boots on! And then he **looked** and saw one his grandchildren was not present.

"Aha!" he said. "You scared me!" He **hugge**d himself tightly and pretended to **shake** in fear. "Don't ever do that again!" *(Tell me about a prank you were involved in either victim or prankster.)*

The children all **danced** inside, including the bear-costumed one. They were **holding their sides laughing hard!** Grandpa **scowled** and **frowned** and then **shrugged his shoulders** and gave each kid **a high-five.**

Grandma saved the day by serving hot chocolate and brownies! They all **ate** with gusto! *(What would that smell like? Taste like?)*

All ended well and the bear suit went into the trunk in the attic FOREVER!

Charlotte Saben, ADC, AP-BC

They had been dubbed "The Three Amigos" but often their wives referred to them more as "The Three Musketeers!" No matter to the guys, they just enjoyed being great friends. Leon and Seth had grown up on the same street, **riding bikes** and causing trouble together. Well, not too much trouble, just a little. They **grinned** at the memories. *(Did you have a nickname when you were younger? Now? What kind of trouble could boys get into?)*

Adam, on the other hand, had lived clear across the nation in a big city and never owned a bike. He **rode** subways instead! He **made a face** at the recollection. But he had found his share of trouble. Like the time he set off a stink bomb on a subway. He still **laughed** about that one…although no one else did. He had never **run so fast** in his life! He probably broke a world's record or something! All the guys **shook their heads** at his tales. *(Did you ever play a prank on someone? Did you get caught? What did a stink bomb smell like? What is your FAVORITE smell?)*

Now they were comparing bucket list adventures! Seth liked to report on all his feats, but Adam and Leon were never quite sure what was true and what was wishful thinking. Leon and Seth had parted ways when Seth went off to college. Leon had stayed behind to run the family business. *(Did you have a family business? Did you go to college?)*

"I already **jumped** out of an airplane," he said, **spreading out his arms** as if floating in air and then **pulling** on a pretend ripcord. He **made circles with his arms** just for good measure. *(Have you parachuted? Did you like it?)*

"Done that plenty of times in the Army!" said Adam. He was quite proud of his service to our country. *(Who has served in the military? THANK YOU!)*

"Well, I also **hiked** the Grand Canyon…in August! Almost died, I did!" He also liked sounding like Yoda from Star Wars. *(Did you see Star Wars movie? What is your favorite movie?)*

"I plan to see ALL Seven Wonders of the World!" said Leon. He **clenched his hands and then opened them** several times. He **pounded one fist into the palm of the other hand.** That meant he was adamant about accomplishing this desire.

Adam began **plucking the air like he was picking cherries,** and **stomping his feet.**

"What are you doing?" asked Seth.

"Well, I always wanted to own a winery; **pick grapes** and make wine all day long!" He **made motions like he was sipping wine**, with his pinky pointing up in snobbish fashion. "But I ended up being an accountant!" He **pouted**.

"Well, you certainly can WHINE all day!" That made them all **bend over** in laughter. Adam pretended to be mad. He **made more faces**. Then he **accentuated his vowels** to avoid actually swearing. The ladies would **frown** about swearing! *(Do you think men should refrain from swearing around ladies Why? Why not?)*

On and on the friends **chatted.** They dreamed of traveling the world, **riding elephants**, **shooting arrows**, **climbing** the highest mountains, and **fishing**…well**, reeling** in the "big catch". They argued over who would get that fish and how they would accomplish it. Of course, Seth was sure it would be him…in fact he already had the fish of record. *(What's the biggest fish you ever caught? Where did you catch it?)*

Adam dreamed of **surfing** in Hawaii. Leon wanted to see in person the Rose Parade on New Year's or the Macy's Thanksgiving Day parade; maybe even **march** alongside a band! He used to play the bass drum. He **flicked his wrists** in memory. Perhaps he could **play a woodwind or trumpet!** He went through all the motions of such. The others **rolled their eyes** and **looked up and down and to the left and right.** Anything to avoid watching his antics! *(Did/Do you play an instrument? In a band?)*

Seth thought trying a zip line across a jungle would satisfy is adventurous spirit. He pretended to **fasten** himself in the harness and **leaned back** for the ride. He **kicked his legs**. He wasn't sure why, but it felt good to be able to do so! *(What do YOU dream of doing? What have you done?)*

The wives **rolled their necks around** in mock disbelief. They **made "chatting" motions** with their fingers and a few other **expressive gestures**.

"Let them dream on!" one of them said. "At least we know where they are!" *(What dreams do you have?)*

Charlotte Saben, ADC, AP-BC

Walter wasn't sure he wanted to go. He **kicked** at the chair in front of him. He knew Gladys wanted him to go, and so did Wayne. Wayne had always been a challenge for Walter. He **swiped at the air** as if his twin brother had gone by. Then he **punched** the air with his fist. Then he **shook his fist** and **accentuated his vowels**. Best to not let Gladys catch him swearing. He knew she would consider it that! Better to make her **roll her eyes** and **shake her head**. *(How do you respond when someone swears?)*

He remembered the duels they had gotten into growing up. He **smiled**. Then he **frowned**. He **rolled his neck** and **breathed deeply**. He might as well **nod his head** and go along with the show. He was no match for Wayne or Gladys. *(Did you and your siblings fight? How? How about your children and grandchildren? Do kids fight differently today than when you were growing up? If yes, how?)*

It was all Wayne's idea! He started up the garage band last month just like he had done in high school. Walter wanted to forget about those days and those antics, but the "others" thought it was a splendid idea! Walter **opened and closed his hands** several times. He wasn't sure they would ever limber up enough to **pluck** those banjo strings again! He practiced air guitar, **strumming** and **tapping his feet**. Yes, those were the days! *(Did you ever play in a band? What kind of music do you like? What is your favorite band?)*

Gladys **walked** into the room and **wiggled her hips slowly**. "How do I look?" she asked expectantly.

Walter wasn't sure what to say. Part of him wanted to **whistle** and part of him wanted to **laugh.** It wasn't that she looked particularly funny…just, well, particular. He **stretched his arms over his head** and **yawned**. It always cleared his brain and bought him some time. *(What is your favorite outfit from your youth?)*

"Well? What do you think?" She was persistent! He **looked to the right and to the left.** Where is that twin brother when you need him? Walter thought almost aloud!

He **looked up and then down**. "Hey! We've got an army of ants **marching** across this floor! I'd better **hop** on down to the basement and get some spray!" Walter had never been so thankful for ants before! *(Do you try to change the subject when something uncomfortable arises? Would you just say she looked nice if you thought differently?)*

Wayne and Norma **knocked** on the door. Walter and Gladys rarely heard the doorbell but could **feel the vibrations** of a **knock**. Norma's attire was equally interesting.

Wayne **bent** to **tuck** his jeans in his boot. He had decades of forgetting that one silly step to looking like a real cowboy. He **flung** his guitar over his shoulder and **reached behind** him to retrieve Walter's old banjo.

"Here ya go, Bro!" he said with a **grin**. "Let's go to the Old Folks Corral and have a show down…I mean a hoe-down! Let's **dance** the night away!"

Gladys disliked the term "Old folks" and **scowled** while **putting her hands on her hips.** "Humph!" she said. "Ya'll can't **play** and **dance** at the same time!" **She moved her hands in the air like she was a ballerina.** *(Did you or your children take ballet lessons?) (Have you been to a ballet? Did you like it? Or do you think you would like it?)*

"Hey! It might turn out to be a showdown after all, Miss Gladys! We ain't playing no fancy ballerina music Girl! You might wanna start the **two-step** or at **least a line dance!** Or have you forgotten how to do that?"

"I was very popular back in our day. My dance card was always full! I **swung** across the floor with most every man in town…I mean, at the dance." *(Did you have a lot of "dates" or suitors when you were younger? What is a dance card?)*

Walter tried not to **laugh** out loud so he **made as many faces** as he could think of. Yep! He had landed the belle of the ball, all right!

The foursome **climbed** up the steps onto the platform, but not as quickly as they had four decades ago…or was it five? Who cares? The band began the familiar music with Norma back on the **drums**. She could still **beat** that skin, her **wrists twisting** only a little bit slower. They songs seemed longer than they used to be, but she **twirled** the sticks in the air nonetheless. *(What is your favorite "Oldie" song? Can you play an instrument?)*

Much to the amazement of Gladys, she still invoked **whistles** and **shouts** from the "young" men…who were much older now. Even the ladies **clapped** and **cheered**. And they joined in. All across the platform ladies dressed in their gingham and pinafores **glided gingerly** together in a line **dance**. The men soon joined as they **waltzed** with their "girls" like there was not a care in the world. *(Do you know how to line dance? Square dance?)*

Gladys **pointed** to the sign which read "Welcome to the Old Folks Corral…where memories are cherished and dreams still come true! And what happens in the corral stays corralled!" Norma **stretched her back** and **hugged** herself and the band members. This had been a good idea after all! And thanks to Kenny who owned the bar for letting those dreams carry on at his "It's Really OK Corral".

Charlotte Saben, ADC, AP-BC

Charlotte Saben, ADC, AP-BC

Charlotte Saben, is certified by the National Certification Council for Activity Professionals (NCCAP) and the National Association of Activity Professionals Credentialing Center (NAAPCC) with over twenty-seven years of experience. She spent much of her time in Skilled Nursing Facilities or Memory Care Units. She has also worked with Assisted Living Residents. Her career started years before that in C.N.A. and R.N.A. positions.

She loves working with seniors and those with physical and mental/emotional challenges. Perhaps this stems from living with her grandparents for most of her formative years. Currently, her challenge has been providing quality opportunities to residents with a broad age span and varied acuity levels. This program was birthed from the need of providing groups for reminiscing, exercising, and experiencing the senses. Combining these components with her love of writing developed into a much-loved program for Seniors in her facility.

Charlotte lives in Surprise, Arizona with her husband and two cattle dog mixes. She is the mother of three grown children and the grandmother of eight.

ACKNOWLEDGEMENTS

I want to thank so many people who have helped make this book a reality. First of all, my husband, Steve Saben, for helping me work through the computer challenges, for assisting with editing, and for believing in me even when I didn't believe in myself!

Rosalind O'Neil, CTRS, ACC, for mentoring and teaching me in so many ways throughout my career; and for specifically encouraging this project.

Diane Mockbee, BS, AC-BC, ACC, for many years of mentoring and teaching by example, and igniting that first spark to get these stories published.

Dale Roberts for teaching, inspiring and basically publishing this book. It would not exist without him.

Rod Bailey for encouraging me and suggesting I meet up with Dale Roberts.

Robert Frechette, Genny Rose, Administrators who believed I could do this!

Many friends and colleagues who inspire me daily.

And most of all: The Residents of LifeStream Complete Senior Living at Sun Ridge, for listening, trying the project, suggesting many topics, and encouraging me to continue writing these stories.